Diabetes
911

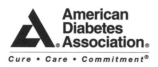

How to Handle
Everyday Emergencies

Larry A. Fox, M.D., and Sandra L. Weber, M.D.

**American
Diabetes
Association**

Cure • Care • Commitment

Director, Book Publishing, Robert Anthony; *Managing Editor, Book Publishing*, Abe Ogden; *Editor*, Greg Guthrie; *Production Manager*, Melissa Sprott; *Composition*, ADA; *Illustrations*, Pam Little, CMI; *Cover Design*, pixiedesign, llc; *Printer*, United Graphics, Inc.

Printed in the United States of America
1 3 5 7 9 10 8 6 4 2

The suggestions and information contained in this publication are generally consistent with the *Clinical Practice Recommendations* and other policies of the American Diabetes Association, but they do not represent the policy or position of the Association or any of its boards or committees. Reasonable steps have been taken to ensure the accuracy of the information presented. However, the American Diabetes Association cannot ensure the safety or efficacy of any product or service described in this publication. Individuals are advised to consult a physician or other appropriate health care professional before undertaking any diet or exercise program or taking any medication referred to in this publication. Professionals must use and apply their own professional judgment, experience, and training and should not rely solely on the information contained in this publication before prescribing any diet, exercise, or medication. The American Diabetes Association—its officers, directors, employees, volunteers, and members—assumes no responsibility or liability for personal or other injury, loss, or damage that may result from the suggestions or information in this publication.

♾ The paper in this publication meets the requirements of the ANSI Standard Z39.48-1992 (permanence of paper).

ADA titles may be purchased for business or promotional use or for special sales. To purchase more than 50 copies of this book at a discount, or for custom editions of this book with your logo, contact the American Diabetes Association at the address below, at booksales@diabetes.org, or by calling 703-299-2046.

American Diabetes Association
1701 North Beauregard Street
Alexandria, Virginia 22311

Library of Congress Cataloging-in-Publication Data

Fox, Larry A.
  Diabetes 911 : how to handle everyday emergencies / by Larry A. Fox and Sandra L. Weber.
    p. cm.
  Includes index.
  ISBN 978-1-58040-300-9 (alk. paper)
  1. Diabetes--Complications. 2. Medical emergencies. I. Weber, Sandra L. II. Title.

RC660.F688 2008
616.4'62025--dc22

2008024026

*This book is dedicated to all of the patients and families
who have taught me so much about diabetes.*

—Larry A. Fox

To my family, with love.

—Sandra L. Weber

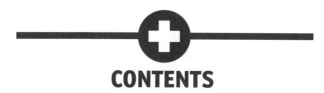

CONTENTS

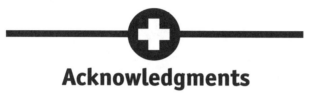

Acknowledgments

I would like to graciously acknowledge the members of the diabetes team and my colleagues and the endocrine staff at Nemours in Jacksonville, all of whom have made immeasurable contributions to the care of children with diabetes. I am especially indebted to Dr. Nelly Mauras, a wonderful friend, colleague, and mentor, whose support over the years has been invaluable.

I am grateful to the American Diabetes Association and its editorial staff for the opportunity to enhance the education and care of patients with diabetes and their families.

Last, but certainly not least, I am forever thankful to my wife, Mary Louise, and my daughters, Erin and Megan, for the endless support and love they have given me.

—Larry A. Fox, M.D.

I wish to thank all who have contributed to a lifetime of learning: my patients, who have shared their joys, frustrations, successes, and struggles; my colleagues, who have provided an environment in which to think and grow; my students, who have kept the desire to learn fresh; and my family, who have always been there, encouraging me to grow and explore and reach.

I am grateful to the American Diabetes Association for their commitment to those with diabetes and to Greg Guthrie for his guidance in preparing this manuscript.

—*Sandra L. Weber, M.D.*

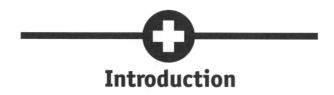

Introduction

People with diabetes have to deal with the same day-to-day emergencies in life as those that occur for people without diabetes. Unfortunately, they also have to deal with a number of diabetes-related emergencies—ones that are not experienced by most people. These include potentially life-threatening events, such as reactions to low blood glucose levels (hypoglycemia) or insulin pump failure, but also include less severe emergencies, such as travel-related diabetes issues. It goes without saying that the best way to deal with any emergency, diabetes-related or not, is to be prepared. That's why we wrote this book.

Diabetes 911 will help you prepare for the emergencies that creep up if you have diabetes. It is a valuable reference for children and adults with diabetes (regardless of whether you have type 1 or type 2). People who are friends or family members of a person with diabetes will also find *Diabetes 911* to be a helpful resource.

Diabetes 911 covers both general emergencies and extreme emergencies. General emergencies are those day-to-day, common pediatric and adult situations. Extreme emergencies are those rare dangerous situations for which you need to be prepared, such as severe weather and power outages. For easy reference, each chapter ends with a summary of its important points.

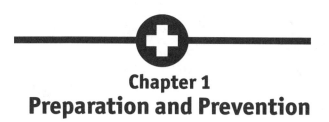

Chapter 1
Preparation and Prevention

People with diabetes experience unique, day-to-day emergencies specific to their condition. Because you have diabetes, you need to be prepared to deal with these emergencies. Alexander Graham Bell, the famous inventor, once said, "Before anything else, preparation is the key to success." Preparing for diabetes emergencies is no exception—*expect the unexpected.* Many diabetes-related problems can be prevented with proper preparation. Here are some beginning steps in preparing for (and hence preventing) a variety of simple but common problems in day-to-day diabetes care.

DIABETES SUPPLY KIT

Scouts are not the only ones who should be prepared. Everyone should. There are many situations when simply having another diabetes supply kit readily available can save you a lot of aggravation and time. Many of these emergencies can be avoided by having

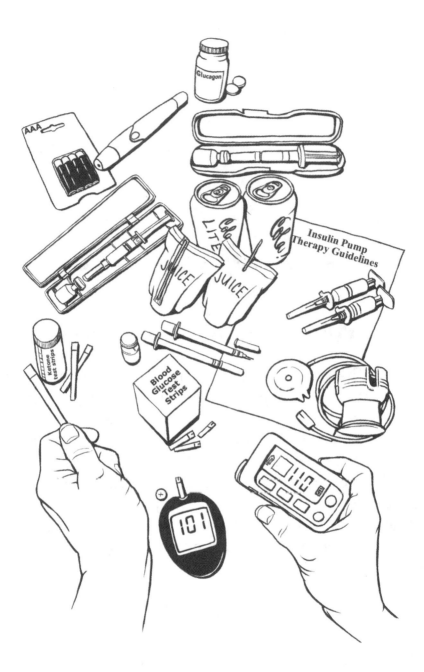

Other Recommendations

EXTRA INSULIN

Bottles of insulin may break when dropped on hard floors. We've had countless calls from frantic patients or parents who need a new insulin prescription called in to the pharmacy because their last vial is now spread across the kitchen floor (and this invariably happens late at night, when most pharmacies are closed). There are many other circumstances in which your time and stress level can be reduced by simply keeping extra insulin available at all times.

PRESCRIPTION REFILLS

Don't wait until the last minute to call your diabetes team for medicine or supply refills. Plan on calling refills in at least one week in advance. You want to be sure that the diabetes team has enough time to review your medical records and take care of your request before you actually run out of insulin, other medicines, or supplies. Remember, diabetes centers treat hundreds—sometimes thousands—of patients and may receive many emergency calls every day. There is no guarantee that they'll be able to get to your request as soon as you need it.

INSULIN PUMP ISSUES

Pump failures can happen, although, luckily, not too commonly. If they do, you may be off your pump for a day or longer. Because the "smart pumps" in use today have the bolus calculations and basal rates programmed into the pump, you may not remember this important information. Avoid being stuck without knowing your insulin doses and keep a written copy of your insulin pump settings, including basal rates, bolus calculations (i.e., meals and high blood glucose boluses), sensitivity factors, target numbers or ranges, and alarms, so pump therapy can be restarted immediately after receiving your replacement. Most insulin pump companies have software that may simplify this process by allowing you to download pump setup information to your home computer. Having this information readily available will make the transition between injections and pump therapy seamless and easy.

Knowing your bolus calculations may also be necessary if you use injections until the pump is replaced. It is also useful to have a vial, cartridge, or pen of long-acting insulin available. The kind and amount of insulin you use should be discussed with your diabetes team, written down, and placed in your diabetes supply kit. For more details about switching to injections while waiting to restart pump therapy, see chapter 4.

SICK DAY SUPPLIES

If you become ill, you'll need extra supplies to ensure that you have a safe and speedy recovery. Make sure that the items for sick day management are at home all the time. If you are vomiting, stay hydrated by taking frequent sips of clear fluids, such as ginger ale, sports drinks, or water (plain or flavored). Popsicles or other frozen fluids are sometimes easier to take in if you are nauseated. Keep both regular and sugar-free fluids on hand: regular for when blood glucose levels are low or in your target range and sugar-free for when you have high blood glucose levels. Be sure your refrigerator or pantry is stocked with these items. You do not want to have to run to the grocery store at the last minute.

Your diabetes team may want you to keep limited amounts of medicines on hand to treat vomiting. Being prepared can help minimize your risks of dehydration and avoid a visit to the emergency room. If your team suggests this, be sure of a few things: 1) the supply is kept up to date (not expired), 2) you know how to use the medicine correctly, and 3) contact your diabetes team before taking the medicine. Also, call or go to the emergency room if, despite the medicine, you are still not able to keep fluids down or your condition worsens.

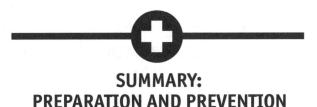

SUMMARY:
PREPARATION AND PREVENTION

YOUR DIABETES SUPPLY KIT INVENTORY

- Diabetes medicines (such as unopened insulin vials and diabetes pills)
- Blood glucose test strips
- Lancets
- Alcohol wipes
- Urine and/or ketone strips
- Items to treat mild or moderate low blood glucose levels (hypoglycemia)
- Glucagon emergency kits (2), if you are at high risk for severe hypoglycemia
- Insulin syringes and/or pen needles
- Extra blood glucose meter and batteries
- Insulin pump supplies—infusion sets, reservoirs, batteries, transparent medical dressings (if used)
- Written instructions from your diabetes team regarding an insulin regimen to follow when off pump therapy (be sure to include the right kind of insulin)

- A list of emergency contact phone numbers for your diabetes team (weekday and evening/weekend numbers), primary care physician, and pharmacy.

YOUR RISK OF SEVERE HYPOGLYCEMIA IS HIGH IF ANY OF THE FOLLOWING APPLY TO YOU

- you are taking insulin or taking a pill that causes your pancreas to make insulin
- you have neuropathy
- you have frequent lows

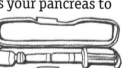

- you cannot recognize the early warning signs of hypoglycemia
- you have had a prior severe low blood glucose reaction

RECOMMENDATIONS FOR HOW YOU CAN LESSEN THE RISK OF SOME COMMON DIABETES PROBLEMS

- Put together a diabetes supply kit and review it monthly. Such a kit should be available at home and in other places where you spend a lot of time (work, school, daycare, and relatives' houses).
- Keep at least one extra bottle or cartridge of insulin available, not only at home but also in other frequented places.
- Give at least one week's notice to your diabetes team or pharmacy when asking for medicine and/or supply refills. For mail-order prescriptions, you may need three weeks.
- Make a backup copy of all insulin pump settings and alarms.

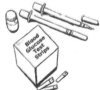

- Keep sick day supplies on hand.

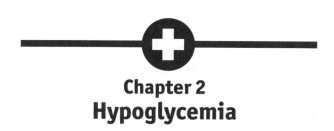

Chapter 2
Hypoglycemia

Hypoglycemia (low blood glucose) is probably the most common emergency in children and adults with diabetes. With the use of more intense insulin regimens, improved blood glucose control comes at the risk of more frequent hypoglycemia. Whether mild, moderate, or severe, hypoglycemia can leave a lasting impression on someone with diabetes or his or her caretaker (especially a parent). In severe cases, hypoglycemia can sometimes have devastating consequences, such as death related to hypoglycemia while driving. Therefore, people with diabetes, and others who spend a lot of time with them (parents, other relatives, school personnel, teachers, co-workers, friends, etc.), need to know how to properly handle this emergency.

This chapter covers recognition and treatment of hypoglycemia. It focuses not only on mild and moderate low blood glucose levels, but also proper treatment of severe events. One of the keys to success with nearly everything is planning ahead—hypoglycemia is no exception. Thus, this chapter also addresses the prevention of hypoglycemia, including when playing sports or exercising. Lastly, this chapter reviews how medications and alcohol influence the development and recognition of hypoglycemia.

SYMPTOMS OF HYPOGLYCEMIA

Hypoglycemia is generally classified as mild, moderate, or severe. This is based on the symptoms of low blood glucose levels (how you feel when your sugar is low). The classification is not based on actual blood glucose numbers. The symptoms of hypoglycemia can vary significantly from person to person and do not entirely depend on the blood glucose level. For example, there can be no symptoms at all, even with a very low blood glucose level (under 40 mg/dl). Or a person can have moderate or severe symptoms with a slightly low blood glucose or a level that is not even low (more than 70 mg/dl).

Many of the symptoms of low blood glucose levels (see sidebar on page 15) are manifestations of the body's response to the low sugar level. Low blood glucose levels activate the sympathetic nervous system, causing early warning signs of hypoglycemia, many of which people recognize. Such symptoms indicate that the body is trying to raise its blood glucose level. These early symptoms are also what you feel when blood glucose drops rapidly but may not be considered low. It is not just the blood glucose level that determines whether someone has symptoms or not—it is also dependent on how fast the blood glucose level is falling.

Other symptoms, however, indicate that the brain is not getting enough of the glucose it needs to function properly. These are the late signs of hypoglycemia and occur if early symptoms are not sensed or recognized or are ignored. The symptoms of mild or moderate hypoglycemia can vary from person to person. Even one person may have different symptoms one day compared with another, depending on surrounding circumstances.

A severe low blood glucose level is much worse and indicates that the brain is severely deprived of the glucose it needs to function properly. Hypoglycemia is always considered severe if it is accompanied by unconsciousness or a seizure (convulsion). It is also severe if you are still conscious but unable to correct the hypoglycemia yourself, whether it is because you cannot recognize it or because you need the help of another person. In infants, toddlers, and young children, this definition does not always apply because they always require someone else's help to treat hypoglycemia, regardless of severity, just by virtue of their young age. It is important to treat severe hypoglycemia immediately to prevent brain damage, but even more important to prevent it altogether.

WHEN DOES HYPOGLYCEMIA OCCUR?

Hypoglycemia occurs when the balance between your insulin levels and the amount of available glucose is disrupted. If your body does not have enough food or is unable to make enough glucose (causing an insufficient amount of glucose available for your body to use for energy), blood glucose levels will decrease. Low blood glucose levels may occur if:

- you skip meals or snacks or eat them much later than usual (if a fixed insulin regimen is used)
- you are not eating enough or eating much less than usual
- you are getting more insulin than you need
- you are getting a lot of exercise or activity
- your liver is unable to make enough glucose

Several diabetes medicines can cause low blood glucose levels, including, of course, insulin. There are other diabetes medicines that can cause relatively high amounts of insulin in the body, which can cause low blood glucose, including a class of drugs called *sulfonylureas*. Examples of sulfonylureas include chlorpropamide (Diabinese), glyburide (Diabeta, Micronase, and others), glipizide (Glucotrol), and glimepiride (Amaryl). Meal-time agents such as Starlix and Prandin have lower risks for hypoglycemia, but still present some risk. Other diabetes medicines generally do not cause hypoglycemia unless they are taken in combination with medications that increase your risk.

A common drug associated with hypoglycemia is *alcohol*. Alcohol has a number of effects that can contribute to low blood glucose levels, and these effects are often delayed up to 12 hours after drinking. Alcohol inhibits the body's defenses against low blood glucose levels: it blocks the liver's ability to make glucose, blocks the effects of chemicals (or *hormones*) in the body that increase glucose production in the liver, blocks the action of insulin (its effectiveness), and impairs your ability to recognize hypoglycemia. Special precautions need to be taken whenever someone with diabetes consumes alcohol. Alcohol consumption and its relation to hypoglycemia are described in depth on page 22.

TREATMENT OF HYPOGLYCEMIA

All low blood glucose levels need to be treated quickly, although the treatment for the different levels of severity (mild or moderate versus severe) varies. If you think you are experiencing hypoglycemia, you should always test your blood glucose level before treating it (unless the low is severe, with unconsciousness or seizure; such cases should be treated before blood glucose is tested).

Mild or Moderate Hypoglycemia

Confirm mild or moderate hypoglycemia with fingerstick testing (under 70 mg/dl). We recommend using the *Rule of 15* to treat mild or moderate hypoglycemia. Treat with 15 grams of carbohydrate; then check the blood glucose level 15 minutes later. Take another

15 grams of carbohydrate if the blood glucose level is not above 70 mg/dl. Depending on a number of factors (such as your actual blood glucose level, plans for exercise, or past experience), you may have to start with 20–30 grams of carbohydrate rather than 15.

AVOID OVERTREATING HYPOGLYCEMIA

This is a common mistake for a few reasons. First, people become nervous about a mild or moderate low turning into a severe one. This is especially true for someone who has experienced a severe low event. It can be very scary, not only for the person with diabetes but also for friends and relatives (especially parents of children with diabetes) who witness the event. Plus, if the severe low is experienced in a public place or at work, it can be very embarrassing. People will do anything to avoid this happening again, including over treatment of low blood glucose or intentionally keeping glucose levels higher than goal.

Second, people have a tendency to treat the symptoms rather

SIGNS OF MILD OR MODERATE HYPOGLYCEMIA

You may feel one or more of the following:

▶ Shaky

▶ Sweaty

▶ Rapid heart beat

▶ Heart palpitations (feeling like your heart is pounding very hard)

▶ Headache

▶ Hungry

▶ Irritable or combative

▶ Tired

▶ Confused

▶ Nervousness or anxiety

▶ Dizzy or lightheaded

---

than the blood glucose level itself. Sometimes the symptoms take a little longer to recover than the blood glucose: blood glucose levels may be back in the target range (or even above it) after treatment, but some of the symptoms will not have disappeared. If this happens, continuing to take carbohydrate will raise blood glucose levels too high. So remember, it is important to treat the blood glucose level, not the symptoms.

Another reason why people overtreat hypoglycemia is because they eat whatever is available without counting carbohydrates. Doing this is much easier than making sure you only get 15 grams of carbohydrate, especially if you are scared, but it can lead to high, fluctuating blood sugars and contributes to poor diabetes control. The overwhelming appetite that accompanies hypoglycemia can sometimes be hard to ignore. Having a plan ahead of time can help control the amount of carbohydrate eaten. An easy solution is to always have a few sources of 15 grams of carbohydrate handy, such as glucose gel or tablets.

Severe Hypoglycemia

The treatment of severe hypoglycemia is different from that for mild or moderate lows. Because the severe low indicates that the brain has very little of the glucose it needs for energy, it is critical to treat these incidents much more aggressively. In these situations, *treat first, ask questions later.*

If the person experiencing severe hypoglycemia is conscious and able to swallow safely, give 30 grams of glucose immediately and

SIGNS OF SEVERE HYPOGLYCEMIA

- Unconsciousness
- Seizure (convulsion)
- Confusion
- Inappropriate conversation/word choice
- Inappropriate behavior
- Sweating

then check his or her blood glucose level. Stay with the person, as the situation may change.

If someone is unconscious or having a seizure, avoid using oral treatments. This person cannot swallow correctly and may suffocate or choke if food or liquids go into the windpipe.

GLUCAGON

Glucagon is used to treat severe lows. Glucagon is a hormone produced by the pancreas that helps the liver make and release glucose into the bloodstream. When injected, glucagon tells the liver to quickly release its stored glucose into the bloodstream. Glucagon comes in small vials or easy-to-use emergency kits. Make sure your close relatives or anyone else with whom you spend a lot of time (spouse, other family members, friends, coworkers, etc.) understands when and how to give a glucagon injection. Your diabetes team can teach anyone how to give glucagon. Glucagon, like insulin, does expire, so you'll need to check the expiration dates for glucagon kits in your diabetes supply kits.

Glucagon is injected into the muscles of the thigh or arm. Adults should use the whole vial (1 mg, or 100 units on an insulin syringe). The amount of glucagon used for children is different than that for adults (see sidebar on page 18 for dosing in infants, toddlers, children, and adolescents). As soon as the glucagon is given, check blood glucose levels, and, if necessary, repeat it in 15 minutes. Be sure to notify your diabetes team of the severe low because changes to your insulin regimen may be required.

If no glucagon is available, call 911 immediately. Glucose gel (or even cake icing) can be used to treat a severe low if glucagon is not available. Squirt the glucose gel or cake icing into the mouth between the cheeks and gums. Carbohydrate is absorbed here, but not as rapidly as desired in an emergency.

Glucagon can also be used in children or adults who have low blood glucose levels and are not able to eat or drink because of vomiting or other reasons. Talk to your diabetes team about using glucagon in these circumstances.

GLUCAGON DOSING FOR CHILDREN AND ADOLESCENTS

The amount of glucagon used for young children and adolescents with diabetes is based on age, as indicated in the chart below, or by weight. Use an insulin syringe to draw up the glucagon and inject it. Talk to your diabetes center for their recommendations on glucagon dosing.

Age	Amount of glucagon
4 years old or younger	0.1 mg (10 units)
5–10 years old	0.2 mg (20 units)
11 years old or older	0.5 mg (50 units)

CALLING 911

There are differing schools of thought regarding if and when to call 911. Some recommend only calling 911 if the glucagon does not work, you cannot find it, or you forget how to use it. Others suggest calling 911 immediately. This way there will not be a delay in the paramedics' arrival if you cannot find the glucagon or if you panic when trying to use it. Talk to your diabetes team about when you should call 911.

PREVENTION OF HYPOGLYCEMIA

Most of the time, with proper planning, hypoglycemia can be prevented. This section covers the prevention of the most frequent causes of low blood glucose levels, including nighttime hypoglycemia and exercise-related hypoglycemia.

Nighttime Hypoglycemia

If you take insulin, one of the most concerning times to have a low blood glucose level is during the night, when you are sleeping. Recent research has shown that a good way to help minimize the chance of nighttime hypoglycemia is to make sure your blood glucose is over 100 mg/dl at bedtime. Before going to sleep, check your blood glucose. If it is under 100 mg/dl, take 15–30 grams of carbohydrate. If a bedtime snack is a part of your self-care regimen and your blood glucose level before the snack was under 100 mg/dl, make sure you check after the snack is finished to be sure that the blood glucose level has risen over 100 mg/dl.

Knowing what your blood glucose level is doing while you are asleep is important. This is especially important for people taking insulin or taking medicines that increase insulin production overnight. We recommend testing blood glucose between bedtime and awakening a couple of times per week, varying the time when the blood glucose check is done. Insulin levels peak at different times; knowing when these peaks occur helps you know the best times to test blood glucose levels. Knowing your blood glucose pattern during your sleep time will guide you in deciding whether any insulin or medicine changes need to be made before low blood glucose levels occur. This will help prevent hypoglycemia (and high blood glucose levels) during sleep hours.

Insulin and Exercise

The important role of exercise in managing diabetes cannot be overemphasized, but with the benefits come the risk of hypoglycemia.

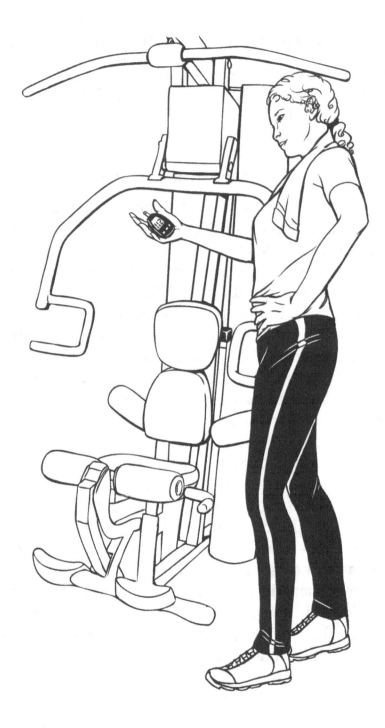

Regular exercise improves the way insulin works in the body and helps you maintain a healthy weight. Exercise also allows the body to use sugar faster, decreasing how much insulin is needed. Thus, exercise can cause hypoglycemia because there is a high amount of insulin in your system relative to the amount of glucose from the liver or from the food you ate. Exercise continues to improve how your body uses glucose, even after you stop exercising. The more frequently and more intensely you exercise, the longer the effects of exercise can last (as long as 24 hours after the activity is over). Therefore, if you are exercising, you may need to take less insulin than usual for up to the next 24 hours.

RECOMMENDATIONS FOR PREVENTING EXERCISE-RELATED HYPOGLYCEMIA

The following recommendations will help minimize the chances of experiencing hypoglycemia related to exercise.

▶ Check your blood glucose before exercising and every 30–60 minutes during the activity, depending on the intensity of the exercise.

▶ You may have to take 15–30 grams of carbohydrate before exercise, depending on your blood glucose level before exercise and the intensity of the exercise you plan to undertake. Experience will tell you what blood glucose levels work best for you before a particular activity. Some people want their blood glucose to be over 100 mg/dl, some over 120 mg/dl, and others over 180 mg/dl before exercising. One recent study in children, however, showed that having a blood glucose level over 130 mg/dl before exercise decreased the chance of experiencing hypoglycemia during exercise. This study was done in children on insulin pumps, so these results may not apply to everyone. Nonetheless, try using 130 mg/dl as a starting level, and if you are below that level, take some extra carbohydrate before exercise. Be sure to talk to your diabetes team for guidance.

▶ Make sure sources of carbohydrate (such as a juice box or glucose tablets or gel) and a glucagon kit are available at all times, including when you are exercising.

- Be sure to check your blood glucose during the activity period. During exercise, if your blood glucose begins to dip below your cutoff point—or if it seems to be dropping quickly—take 15–30 grams of carbohydrate. Recheck your blood glucose level 15 minutes later to be sure it has not dropped further.

- Insulin dose changes may be required during the activity and possibly even later, because the effects of exercise on insulin needs can last up to 24 hours.

- If you use an insulin pump, changes in your basal rates may be required. Many people disconnect their pump before starting exercise. Some research has shown that hypoglycemia is much less likely during exercise if the basal rate is stopped. However, we recommend not being disconnected from your insulin pump for more than two hours at a time because this may leave the body without insulin for too long. You can also decrease your basal rate through your insulin pump using the temporary basal rate features. Talk to your diabetes team about changes to your insulin pump regimen during and after exercise.

Knowing your needs and your response to exercise is critical. Different exercise routines, regimens, or even times of day can give very different responses. The key is to be proactive and learn your patterns by monitoring, reviewing, and adjusting to your needs.

As a reminder, the effects of exercise on insulin needs can last up to 24 hours after the exercise is over. Because of this, it is not uncommon to experience hypoglycemia in the middle of the night after a day of activity. This is obviously a time when lows need to be prevented. Be sure to check blood glucose levels frequently after exercising, including during late night or early morning hours.

Alcohol

Several precautions need to be taken when it comes to having diabetes and drinking alcohol (see sidebar on page 24). Alcoholic beverages can contain carbohydrate and may cause blood glucose levels to

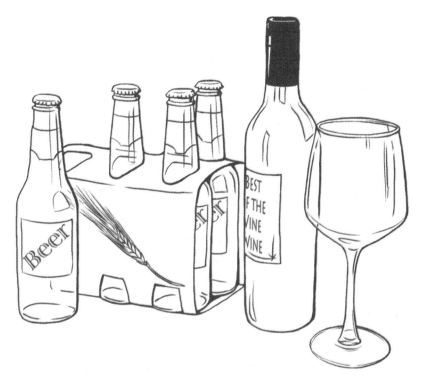

initially rise. However, alcohol impairs the body's response to low or decreasing blood glucose levels. This effect can be quite delayed, up to 12 hours after drinking. Additionally, alcohol impairs judgment, so your ability to recognize and treat hypoglycemia will be reduced. When slightly intoxicated or drunk your ability to think straight is altered; you may not recognize hypoglycemia when it happens and may not treat it properly even if you do. Alcohol is metabolized (broken down) by the liver, and during this process, the liver does not make as much glucose as normal. Thus, alcohol impairs one of the body's key responses to low blood glucose—releasing stored glucose from the liver to raise blood glucose levels.

Food-Related Hypoglycemia

Skipping a meal, eating late, or eating less than expected can cause hypoglycemia. There are countless situations in which this can happen. This can occur if you are sick, when most people don't feel well and have less of an appetite. If you're still taking the same amount of insulin (or other medications that lower blood glucose) and eat fewer carbohydrates than usual, then low blood glucose may occur. If you have lost your appetite, it may help to take carbohydrate in fluid form rather than as solid food, especially if you are experiencing vomiting. Chapter 3 covers sick day management in more detail.

Another common situation arises in people who use multiple daily injections or an insulin pump. With these regimens a dose of rapid-acting insulin is calculated based on the amount of carbohydrate to be consumed. If the insulin dose is given for a certain amount of carbohydrate (for example, 75 grams) but less is actually eaten (for example, only 60 grams), then hypoglycemia may occur because of the extra insulin given. This is sometimes unavoidable. If it occurs, one solution to prevent hypoglycemia is to drink the amount of carbohydrate not consumed (in our example above, 15 grams). In general, it is best to err on the low side when it comes to counting carbohydrates. If you are not sure if you're going to eat something and you are choosing between 60 and 75 grams because of it, then be conservative—bolus for the 60 grams. If you do not eat the item, you are fine. If you do eat the extra 15 grams, you can bolus for it later.

Insulin Errors

Mistakes happen. After all, we are human. Even people who have had diabetes for many years occasionally make mistakes with insulin dosing. Most of the time, mistakes occur because people are in a hurry. One way to help prevent these mistakes is to confirm your dose with someone else (a spouse or parent, for example) before giving it. This includes not only reviewing the dose and calculations, but also confirming that the right dose is drawn up into the syringe and the correct type of insulin is taken. Insulin pens make some of these dosing errors less likely.

Taking the wrong insulins at the wrong time—or reversing insulin doses—is another common mistake. For example, the higher morning dose of NPH is taken instead of the lower evening or bedtime dose. In this scenario, the higher dose of insulin in the evening leads to low blood glucose levels in the late night and early morning hours. If this happens, the only reasonable solution is to eat extra carbohydrate and to frequently check your blood glucose levels throughout the night. If you live alone it is important to have a backup system in place if you reverse your insulin doses; for example, someone who can come over or check on you during the night or be a contact to call at regular intervals. Be sure to contact your diabetes team for help if this happens to you and your blood glucose levels are decreasing.

On occasion, rapid-acting insulin (such as insulin aspart [Novo-Log], insulin lispro [Humalog], or insulin glulisine [Apidra]) is taken instead of long-acting insulin (insulin glargine [Lantus] or insulin detemir [Levemir]). Although the vials of these rapid-acting insulins look different from the long-acting ones, they are all clear insulin and can be easily confused, especially if you are in a hurry. Again, the best way to prevent this is by double checking your doses and having someone else recheck everything for you. Should this mistake occur, the only way to prevent a low is to take in additional carbohydrate and check your blood glucose levels often. Contact your diabetes team for help with this situation.

Continuous Glucose Monitors

The ability to monitor glucose levels much more frequently, as often as every minute, is a valuable option for the prevention of hypoglycemia and as an alternate means of recognizing hypoglycemia. This is a relatively new technology in the market but several products are available. Continuous glucose monitors check interstitial glucose levels from a site placed in the subcutaneous tissue (just below the skin). A continuous glucose monitor does not give the same glucose reading as a blood glucose level, but they are very good for looking at trends, including anticipation of hypoglycemia. The devices have different alarms and/or visual signals to notify a person of gradual or rapid decrease (or rise) in the blood glucose level. This can be a lifesaving device for someone who cannot recognize hypoglycemia or who has widely fluctuating levels.

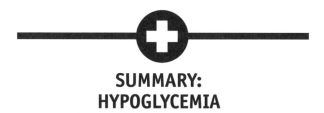

SUMMARY:
HYPOGLYCEMIA

SIGNS OF MILD OR MODERATE HYPOGLYCEMIA

You may feel one or more of the following:

- Shaky
- Sweaty
- Rapid heart beat
- Heart palpitations (feeling like your heart is pounding very hard)
- Headache
- Hungry
- Irritable or combative
- Tired
- Confused
- Nervousness or anxiety
- Dizzy or lightheaded

HYPOGLYCEMIA MAY OCCUR IF:

- You skip meals or snacks or eat them much later than usual (if a fixed insulin regimen is used)
- You are not eating enough or eating much less than usual
- You are getting more insulin than you need
- You are getting a lot of exercise or activity
- Your liver is unable to make enough glucose

THE RULE OF 15: AFTER CONFIRMING THAT THE BLOOD GLUCOSE IS LOW VIA FINGERSTICK:

- Give 15 grams of carbohydrate (e.g., 4 ounces juice, 3–4 glucose tablets, or 4 ounces regular soda).

- Recheck blood glucose 15 minutes later.
- Repeat process until blood glucose is over 70 mg/dl.

**GLUCAGON DOSING FOR
CHILDREN AND ADOLESCENTS:**

The amount of glucagon used for young children and adolescents with diabetes is based on age or weight, as indicated in the chart below. Use an insulin syringe to draw up the glucagon and inject it.

Age	Amount of glucagon
4 years old or younger	0.1 mg (10 units)
5–10 years old	0.2 mg (20 units)
11 years old or older	0.5 mg (50 units)

PREVENTING EXERCISE-RELATED HYPOGLYCEMIA

- Check your blood glucose levels frequently (including before, during, and after exercise).
- If you use insulin, make any necessary insulin adjustments. If you are on an insulin pump, this includes possibly disconnecting from the pump during exercise (or suspending or using temporary basal rates).
- Take extra carbohydrate before the activity if your blood glucose is below your cutoff (for example, 130 mg/dl).
- Make sure juice boxes, glucose tablets or gel, or other forms of carbohydrate and glucagon are available at all times, even while active.
- Remember that the effects of exercise on insulin requirements can last for up to 24 hours after the period of exercise is over. Because of this, your insulin needs may be lower after the exercise is over.

PREVENTING ALCOHOL-RELATED HYPOGLYCEMIA

▶ Be sure to eat whenever you consume alcohol.

▶ If you are on multiple daily injections or use an insulin pump, bolus for the carbohydrate eaten or in drink mixers but NOT for the carbohydrate in the alcohol.

▶ Have a bedtime snack before you go to sleep after drinking.

▶ Don't sleep in; wake up at your usual time and check your blood glucose.

▶ Drink in moderation and, of course, do not drink and drive.

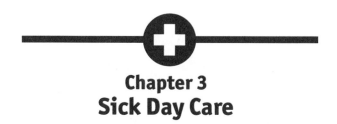

Chapter 3
Sick Day Care

Everyone gets sick at some point. Most of the time it can be dealt with at home, but knowing what to do and when to go to the emergency room is important.

DEALING WITH ILLNESS

Getting sick is never fun. With diabetes, you also have to consider many more issues—you have to think like a pancreas. If you are sick, your body normally makes "stress hormones" to deal with illness. Stress hormones change how the body uses insulin, making it more resistant to insulin's effects. More insulin resistance means the body needs more insulin to get the same glucose response, and the pancreas would normally respond by making more insulin. Insulin requirements can therefore be very high during illness and, depending on how much insulin your pancreas is able to make, an illness can cause you to require more insulin than your body can produce. Whether or not you are taking insulin, these higher insulin needs have to be addressed. This can be

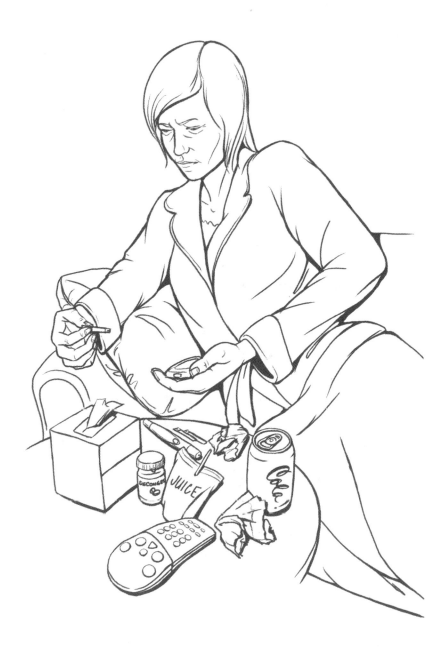

accomplished by taking insulin (or increasing your doses, if you are already on insulin), stimulating insulin release (through oral medications), or modifying your glucose intake (adjusting how much food or drink you take in). In addition to your increased need for insulin, you'll also need to take in calories and stay hydrated, so you can get healthy. During illness, as in daily life, you need to balance fluids, food, and medication needs.

Keeping the right amount of fluids in your body is important for everyone who gets sick. It is often best to frequently drink small amounts of fluid, sipping as often as possible. Drinking larger volumes can sometimes trigger nausea and vomiting. There is no specific recommended beverage when nausea and vomiting are a problem—you will usually know what doesn't make you sick. If it is hard to drink fluids, frozen items are sometimes better tolerated. Popsicles or other frozen fruit pops (either commercially available or homemade from juices or drinks) and other similar items are great to have in your freezer for a sick day when vomiting is a problem.

Should you have fluids that contain sugar? If you are not able to eat solid food and drinking is your only option, then you should drink fluids with sugar. If you drink only water, you will not get any calories. This can make sickness worse, especially after being ill for 24 hours. Calorie needs can be higher than usual during illness. If your blood glucose levels are very high, however, taking in more sugar will make things worse. The best thing to do is to monitor your blood glucose frequently, take medicines to deal with your blood glucose levels, and drink glucose-containing fluids, unless your blood glucose levels are high.

Should you have other nutrients in your liquids? This depends on what the rest of your body is doing. If you have a fever, vomiting, or diarrhea, you are losing electrolytes (the salts in the body) in addition to the fluids. In these situations, it is important to replace the salts, too. Sports drinks

WHAT TO DRINK WHEN YOU'RE SICK

▶ Water

▶ Sugar-containing fluids (especially clear liquids, such as lemon-lime soda, ginger ale, fruit juice, etc.)

▶ Sports drinks

▶ Pedialyte (generally for infants and toddlers)

or specific sick-day drinks, such as Pedialyte (for infants and possibly toddlers), have these salts in them and are good choices. Remember that many of these drinks have sugar, too, but many newer products exist that are very low in carbohydrates, 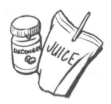 such as Propel or Gatorade's G2 product line. Those that do contain carbohydrate should be avoided if blood glucose levels are high. Children, especially infants and toddlers, can lose large amounts of fluids and electrolytes quickly, so it is important to have electrolyte-containing fluids in your sick day kit (see sidebar below).

If you are not able to eat or drink anything, your condition will probably get worse. Because the goal is to at least keep drinking fluids, keeping nausea and vomiting under control is important. Anti-nausea medications can be very helpful in this situation. There are several medications available that come in pill, suppository, and injectable forms. These should be in your sick day kit. Discuss with your doctor ahead of time which anti-nausea medication is best for you and how to use it correctly. Be sure to contact your diabetes team if you have any questions or if you are not improving. If you have vomiting that cannot be controlled and you cannot keep any fluids down, you need to go to an emergency

SICK DAY KIT INVENTORY

▶ Blood glucose test strips

▶ Urine and/or blood ketone test strips

▶ Fluids to drink (some with and some without sugar)

▶ Frozen fruit pops or other similar frozen items

▶ Anti-nausea medications (pills and/or suppositories)

▶ A list of emergency contact phone numbers (your diabetes team [weekday and evening/weekend numbers], primary care physician, and pharmacy)

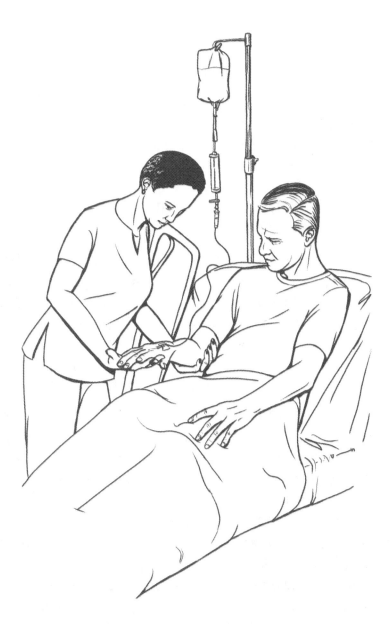

facility so intravenous fluids and medicines can be given. If you are losing more fluids than you can take in, you should also seek emergency care.

Your stomach is controlled by nerves, and the timing of these nerves is easily disturbed when you are sick. In addition, some people have *diabetic neuropathy* (nerve damage caused by years of high blood glucose levels). If neuropathy affects the stomach, it is called *gastroparesis*. People who have gastroparesis have problems with the timing of food mixing in the stomach and emptying from it. Gastroparesis typically gets worse during an illness. Gastroparesis is associated with early, severe, and frequent nausea and vomiting. Medicines that deal with gastroparesis are available, and you should discuss this with your diabetes team if you need them.

MONITORING BLOOD GLUCOSE LEVELS AND KETONES

With diabetes and illness, you need information! Remember, you need to think like a pancreas and that means you need to know what your blood glucose level is, how it is changing, and how you should respond. Monitoring is even more important when you are sick. You need to know your body's extra needs.

How Often Should You Monitor When Sick?

If you are not on insulin, you need to know if your pancreas is making enough insulin in response to the illness. You may need to check your blood glucose levels at least two to four times a day. If your blood glucose levels are in the normal range, checking twice a day should be adequate. If your levels are consistently high, then you need more medicine. Discuss with your diabetes team whether this means adding or taking more of an insulin-stimulating medicine or starting insulin.

If you are already on insulin, then you need to know how much more insulin you need and when. It is important to monitor blood glucose levels before and after eating to see if you are meeting the higher basal and meal insulin needs that come with being sick. You want to be able to correct high glucose levels with insulin if they arise, so plan on monitoring your levels at least every four hours. The amount of additional insulin may be the same as your usual supplemental dose, or it could be higher, depending on your previous experiences with illness. Discuss using supplemental insulin with your diabetes team. The presence or absence of ketones (see *Monitoring ketones* below) can help guide you in determining your insulin needs. If you have moderate or large urine ketones—or high blood ketones—then you have increased insulin (and fluid) needs. If this happens to you, insulin doses should be increased by about 10%. Talk to your diabetes team for specific changes to your insulin doses if you have moderate or large ketones.

Monitoring should be consistently done at designated times throughout the illness. It is important to have an accurate blood glucose meter and enough testing supplies (lancets, strips, etc.) for higher sick-day monitoring needs. Continuous glucose monitors are also available and can be useful during sickness. Continuous glucose monitors track blood glucose trends by frequently checking blood glucose levels (up to every minute). Some of these devices can also be used with an insulin pump. However, remember that a continuous glucose monitor still requires fingerstick blood glucose monitoring to make sure that the blood and interstitial glucose levels are correlating. When glucose levels are varying a lot, as they may during an illness, it is a good idea to confirm more often.

MONITORING KETONES

Ketones develop when the body has to use something other than glucose for energy and usually occur when the body breaks down fat for energy. Small amounts of ketones are common in the body when you are not eating or when you first wake up (especially in young children). But if ketone levels in urine or blood are high or rising, then this is a clue that more intensive treatment is needed. High or rising ketone levels are typically seen in people with little to no insulin production, worsening illness, and relatively too little insulin in the bloodstream for their body's needs (which, remember, are often higher during illness). *Generally, people with diabetes should check for ketones when they are sick or when blood glucose levels are high (over 250 mg/dl).* Ketones are less common in people with type 2 diabetes, but they can still occur. There are monitoring strips that check for ketones in the urine, and some blood glucose meters can check for ketones in the blood.

The presence of moderate or large amounts of urine or blood ketones indicates that the body lacks enough insulin. Because the body requires more insulin during illness, moderate or large amounts of blood or urine ketones indicate that these needs are not being met. The presence of ketones tells you that more aggressive insulin and fluid treatments need to be undertaken quickly. If left untreated, high amounts of ketones can lead to *diabetic ketoacidosis*, a very dangerous condition (see sidebar on page 39).

DIABETES MEDICINES DURING ILLNESS

There are a few basic concepts that need to be understood when dealing with diabetes medicines and illnesses. First, illness is a stress to the body, and any source of stress increases insulin resistance. When insulin resistance is higher, you need more insulin to get the same effect on blood glucose levels.

Second, your body always needs insulin for different jobs. The body uses insulin to control many things: how the liver makes glucose, how energy is stored as fat, and much more. Insulin allows your body to get the energy you need from the food you eat. Insulin requirements change, and the amount of insulin your body requires changes a lot when you are sick. Even more insulin will be needed to cover the food you eat and to correct high glucose levels during illness.

Third, the most important concept to understand is that in people without diabetes, the pancreas continuously makes insulin—24 hours a day. So, even when you are sick and not eating, your body still needs insulin. *This is very important.* Many people make the common mistake of thinking that they do not need insulin when

DIABETIC KETOACIDOSIS

Diabetic ketoacidosis (or DKA) is a potentially life-threatening condition and a serious medical emergency. DKA arises from a combination of too little insulin and high levels of stress hormones. If your pancreas is making little or no basal insulin, it is *critical* that you continue taking basal insulin. DKA can occur in people with either type 1 or type 2 diabetes, but it is more common in people with type 1 diabetes.

DKA requires immediate care in the hospital, so get help if you begin to develop the symptoms of DKA. It usually develops slowly. But when vomiting occurs, it can develop within a few hours.

THE FIRST SYMPTOMS ARE

▶ Thirst or a very dry mouth

▶ Frequent urination

▶ High blood glucose levels (over 250 mg/dl)

▶ High levels of urine ketones

NEXT, OTHER SYMPTOMS APPEAR

▶ Constantly feeling tired

▶ Dry or flushed skin

▶ Nausea, vomiting, or abdominal pain (Vomiting can be caused by many illnesses, not just ketoacidosis. If vomiting continues for more than two hours, contact your health care provider.)

▶ A hard time breathing (short, deep breaths)

▶ Fruity odor on the breath

▶ A hard time paying attention or confusion

they are sick because they are not eating. *The body always needs insulin to perform its other duties.* If you take insulin, your dose may need to be changed, but you still need to take some insulin, even during the worst illnesses. If you take pills to increase your insulin production, keep taking them.

Insulin Pump Therapy

Insulin pumps are designed to deal with varying insulin requirements. They have separate settings for basal, meal bolus, and correction doses to meet different insulin needs. The basal insulin setting delivers a constant dose of insulin to the body. If you are sick, you still need basal insulin, whether you are eating or not. The meal bolus insulin setting deals with the amount of carbohydrate you will eat and is usually taken before eating. If you are sick and unsure that you'll be able to keep down food (i.e., you've been vomiting), it may be safer to take your bolus after you have eaten and are confident that you won't vomit. Use your judgment.

The cornerstone of diabetes care during sickness is correction insulin. Because your body is rapidly changing its insulin needs, you need frequent information to decide how much insulin to take. Check your blood glucose levels every four hours or as recommended by your diabetes team and take correction doses as needed (but no more than every two hours) until you are healthy again. Once you are healthy, resume your usual routine.

Insulin Injections

Different insulins have different times in which they achieve peak effectiveness. Discuss how to adjust these insulins during illness with your diabetes team ahead of time so you are prepared and do not have to figure it out when you are sick. When using multiple injection (or basal-bolus) therapy, the long-acting insulins (insulin glargine [Lantus] and insulin detemir [Levemir]) provide your basal (or background) insulin needs. That part of your insulin regimen should be continued when you are sick. However, the amount of rapid-acting insulin (insulin lispro [Humalog], insulin aspart [NovoLog], and insulin glulisine [Apidra]), and sometimes regular insulin, that you take for meals may have to be adjusted. The adjustments for people who use NPH insulin are more challenging because it has a significant peak effectiveness that can be variable. If you are sick, your diabetes team may recommend that you reduce your dose of NPH insulin by one-third to one-half. If you use a premixed insulin (e.g., 70/30, 75/25, or 50/50), it is recommended to cut the dose in half, but check with your diabetes team first. Discuss all of these issues beforehand and have your sick care plan written down. Proper preparation will keep you from making insulin mistakes when you are ill.

Diabetes Pills

Diabetes pills are hard to take when you are nauseated and vomiting. If you can control the nausea with anti-nausea medicines, it is a good idea to continue taking your diabetes medicines. The exception to this rule is metformin (Glucophage): if you cannot keep fluids down, you may lose a lot of fluids and possibly hurt your kidneys. Do not take metformin until you are sure that you are able to eat and drink.

If you are not able to keep anything down, you will not be able to take your diabetes pills. If this happens to you, you need to have a backup plan ready. Discuss options with your diabetes team beforehand to decide what to do in a situation like this. You will have to work together to determine a blood glucose level cutoff, above which you need to call your diabetes team to put the backup plan into action. Sometimes, this will mean that you will have to take insulin for a short while, until you are healthy again. Be sure to contact your diabetes team for help with managing your diabetes pills during an illness.

WHEN TO GO TO THE EMERGENCY ROOM

Usually, you'll know when to go to the emergency room for additional care, but sometimes when you are sick, you can't make that decision on your own. If you cannot keep any fluids down, go to the emergency room immediately. If you can drink enough fluids and maintain pretty good blood glucose control, keep up with what you're doing, but keep a close eye on your blood glucose levels. Other serious situations will require quick action and an immediate trip to the emergency room (see sidebar below). Don't forget that there is usually a reason why you are sick in the first place and that may also need treatment. Always err on the side of caution! If you are not sure whether a trip to the emergency room is necessary, call your diabetes team for guidance.

WHEN TO GO TO THE EMERGENCY ROOM

Seek immediate help if any of the following apply to you.

- You are unable to keep down any fluids (vomiting) or losing a lot of fluid (diarrhea or sweating)
- Signs of diabetic ketoacidosis, such as rapid breathing, fruity breath, etc. (see sidebar on page 39)
- Constantly high blood glucose levels (usually above 250 mg/dl)
- Large (or rising) amounts of urine or blood ketones
- Another illness (such as the flu) that needs attention

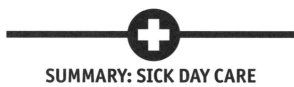

SUMMARY: SICK DAY CARE

WHAT TO DRINK WHEN YOU'RE SICK
- Water
- Sugar-containing fluids (especially clear liquids, such as lemon-lime soda, ginger ale, fruit juice, etc.)
- Sports drinks
- Pedialyte (generally for infants and toddlers)

SICK DAY KIT INVENTORY
- Blood glucose test strips
- Urine and/or blood ketone strips
- Fluids to drink (some with and some without sugar)
- Frozen fruit pops or other similar frozen items
- Anti-nausea medications (pills and/or suppositories)
- A list of emergency contact phone numbers (your diabetes team [weekday and evening/weekend numbers], primary care physician, and pharmacy)

DIABETIC KETOACIDOSIS
The first symptoms are
- Thirst or a very dry mouth
- Frequent urination
- High blood glucose levels (over 250 mg/dl)
- High levels of urine ketones

Next, other symptoms appear
- Constantly feeling tired
- Dry or flushed skin
- Nausea, vomiting, or abdominal pain (Vomiting can be caused by

many illnesses, not just ketoacidosis. If vomiting continues for more than two hours, contact your health care provider.)

- A hard time breathing (short, deep breaths)
- Fruity odor on the breath
- A hard time paying attention or confusion

WHEN TO GO TO THE EMERGENCY ROOM

Seek immediate help if any of the following apply to you.

- You are unable to keep down any fluids (vomiting) or losing a lot of fluid (diarrhea or sweating)
- Signs of diabetic ketoacidosis, such as rapid breathing, fruity breath, etc. (see sidebar on page 39)
- Constantly high blood glucose levels (usually above 250 mg/dl)
- Large (or rising) amounts of urine or blood ketones
- Another illness (such as the flu) that needs attention

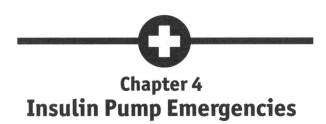

Chapter 4
Insulin Pump Emergencies

Intensive insulin therapy is the practice of rigorously using insulin therapy to achieve blood glucose levels in the nondiabetic range. It has become the goal for many adults and children with type 1 diabetes and is often achieved by using an insulin pump. Because of this popular goal, the number of people with either type 1 or type 2 diabetes who are changing to insulin pump therapy has been increasing over the past several years. Scientific research has clearly shown that excellent diabetes control helps limit or prevent diabetes complications. Strict control of blood glucose levels also offers people with diabetes an improved lifestyle. But with these advantages come some risks.

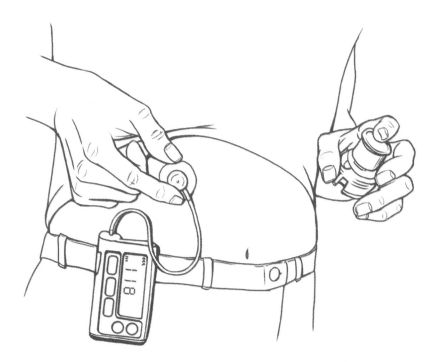

Many people who are on an intensive insulin therapy regimen use an insulin pump, and, as with any mechanical device, insulin pumps can break and seem to do so at the worst times (not that there is ever a *good* time). When an insulin pump fails, the loss of insulin can occur quickly, potentially leading to diabetic ketoacidosis (DKA; see page 39). If your insulin pump breaks, you must use insulin injections while waiting for a replacement pump. This can sometimes take days. People with diabetes and their families should be prepared for these situations and educated on how to deal with them.

An important word of caution: this information should be used as a guideline. Be sure to contact your diabetes team for specific insulin recommendations.

PREPARATION

Thus far we have repeatedly emphasized the importance of anticipating potential problems. Being prepared for pump problems is no exception—a significant amount of trouble can be avoided if you anticipate pump problems and have made proper preparations. You'll want to put together a pump supply kit to be ready for problems (see sidebar below).

INTERRUPTED INSULIN DELIVERY

Insulin pumps provide a continuous supply of insulin (the *basal* or *background rate*) throughout the day and night. This is intended to mimic your own body's insulin release, which in people without diabetes never goes to zero. Even at night, when you are not eat-

---

PUMP SUPPLY KIT INVENTORY

▶ Make two lists of all pump settings, including doses for meal boluses, high blood glucose boluses, and all basal rates and patterns. The lists should also include your target blood glucose levels, target ranges, etc. Some pump manufacturers allow you to download these settings to your home computer (or even to the manufacturer's online service over the Internet). This is a good way to keep a backup of your pump settings. Keep one list separate from the rest of your pump supply kit (in case you lose the pump supply kit).

▶ Be sure to have an adequate supply of rapid-acting insulin pens and pen needles available. If you use insulin syringes, be sure to have an adequate supply of them as well as insulin vials for day-to-day pump use.

▶ Keep some long-acting insulin pens or vials (e.g., insulin glargine [Lantus] or insulin detemir [Levemir]) available. The long-acting insulin may be used if injections are needed while waiting for a replacement pump.

▶ Keep extra pump batteries available at all times.

▶ Keep two or more extra infusion sets and related supplies.

ing, your pancreas still continues to make and release some insulin. If insulin delivery from your pump stops, the basal insulin will be used fairly quickly, lasting only a few hours (insulin analogs, such as insulin glulisine [Apidra], insulin aspart [NovoLog], and insulin lispro [Humalog], are used this fast; regular insulin may last longer). After a short amount of time the body will not be getting any insulin.

If this happens, you will need to take rapid-acting insulin because your body would otherwise be without insulin. You will also have to figure out what has caused the delivery of insulin to be disrupted. The sidebar above describes some of the common causes of interrupted insulin delivery. Sometimes the cause of the problem is obvious, but other times some detective work is necessary.

Pump Malfunctions

Simply put, insulin pumps can break, just like any other mechanical device, even though they have few moving parts. The good news, however, is that all pumps are programmed to sound an alarm when something is wrong with the pump itself. Each pump has its own array of alarm codes and meanings, so be sure to review your insulin pump manual periodically, so you are prepared.

If your pump is indicating that there is a problem, take it seriously. It can be easy to silence the alarm and forget about it, but this can potentially lead to serious problems, such as DKA, that could have been avoided. Depending on the alarm, you might be able to easily remedy the problem yourself. Sometimes it takes a

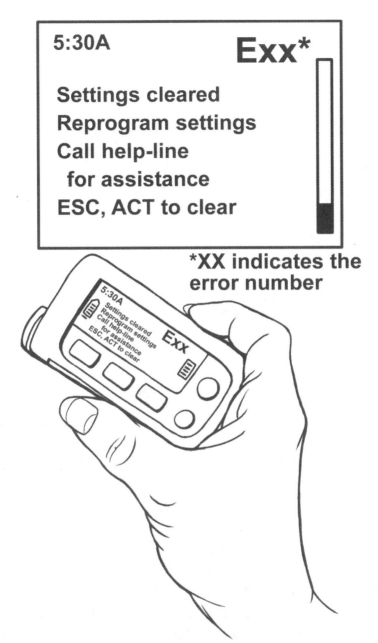

5:30A   Exx*

Settings cleared
Reprogram settings
Call help-line
  for assistance
ESC, ACT to clear

*XX indicates the
error number

call to the manufacturer to help decipher the code and trouble-shoot the problem. Also, be sure to call your diabetes team if the pump is not working—they may be able to help or they may have to guide you with insulin doses if changes are needed.

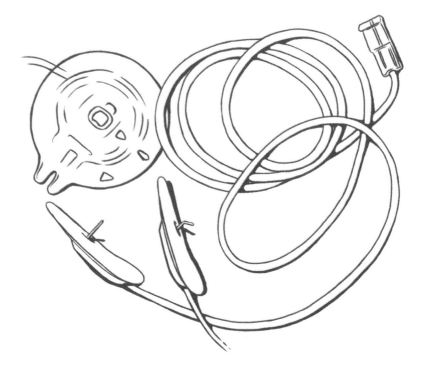

Catheter Problems

If you are experiencing steady, unexplained increases in blood glucose levels that do not respond to the usual boluses used to correct high blood glucose levels, you may have an insulin delivery problem, the most common of which are kinks in the tubing (the part that leads from the reservoir to the cannula) or in the cannula (the part that goes just under the skin). Visually inspect the following for problems: the insulin pump, the connection with the reservoir, the tubing, the connection with the cannula, and the cannula itself. The system up to the connection with the cannula can also be tested by disconnecting the tubing from the cannula, giving a test bolus, and watching to see if there is insulin delivery. Insulin delivery problems can be serious. A person can develop DKA if he or she does not notice that the insulin pump is not delivering insulin for several hours, such as while sleeping overnight. If DKA is developing, your blood glucose level will be very high and you will have moderate or large amounts of urine or blood ketones. The signs of DKA are described on page 39.

The sidebar below lists the general guidelines for managing pump problems. One common mistake is for people to keep giving boluses through the pump to correct high blood sugars, even though the sugars are not responding to the boluses (i.e., the blood glucose level has not decreased or has increased). Only give one high blood glucose bolus with the pump; if there is no response to that bolus within two hours, an insulin injection needs to be given and the pump infusion set should be changed. This may be the only way you will know if the infusion set cannula is kinked—by *looking at it* after changing the site.

GUIDELINES FOR PUMP PROBLEMS

When pump problems occur, follow these general guidelines.

▶ You may need to check your blood glucose more often than usual, sometimes as often as every two hours.

▶ Check the pump, catheter tubing, and infusion site for obvious problems.

▶ If the cannula is out, insert a new infusion set and give a high blood glucose bolus using the pump and your usual correction dose.

▶ Check your urine (or blood, if possible with your meter) for ketones when blood glucose levels are over 250 mg/dl. You will need more insulin if moderate or large amounts of urine ketones are present. Continue to check ketones. This can be useful in determining whether your situation is getting better or worse.

▶ *Only give one high blood glucose bolus with the pump.* If there is no response to that bolus (i.e., your blood glucose level has not changed or has increased) within two hours, an insulin injection needs to be given.

Fixing Insulin Pump Problems

If your pump sounds an alarm and you can't immediately tell what is wrong, look at the pump manual for guidance. If you cannot solve the pump problem yourself, call the pump manufacturer. All pump companies have a 24-hour toll-free number located on the pump. The support staff will help you troubleshoot problems. If the problem cannot be fixed over the phone, arrangements will be made for sending you a replacement pump. If this happens to you, you will have to use insulin injections until the new pump arrives. Details on a temporary insulin injection regimen are described below.

TEMPORARY INSULIN REGIMEN

If you cannot fix your insulin pump on your own, the pump manufacturer will send you a new one using overnight delivery. In some cases, if this happens on a Friday or over a holiday, the replacement pump may not arrive until two or even three days later. Sometimes, a local sales representative for the pump company may be able to get you a temporary pump, but even this may take several hours. While waiting for the replacement pump—whether it takes only several hours or a number of days—you will have to go back on insulin injections until the pump arrives. If the new pump is expected to arrive within a few hours (and not overnight), figuring out the proper insulin doses is easy—injections for only high blood glucose levels and meal boluses will be required. Thus, you can use the same doses and same insulin as you use with your pump (probably a rapid-acting insulin), but by injecting it instead.

Which Insulin?

If it will take more than a few hours or overnight to get your replacement pump, managing insulin is a little trickier. Some people choose to only use rapid-acting insulin until the pump is replaced. The disadvantage of this decision is that insulin injections will be required every four to six hours, including overnight, because

Guidelines for a Temporary Insulin Regimen

▶ Try contacting the pump manufacturer's local sales representative to get a replacement pump immediately rather than waiting for one to be shipped to you.

▶ *If you have a short wait for your replacement pump.* You can use rapid-acting insulin only (using your usual meal and correction bolus doses), but this requires injections every four to six hours. This is often not a problem during the day but can be inconvenient at night.

▶ *If you have a long wait for your replacement pump (24 hours or longer).* Long-acting insulin, such as insulin detemir (Levemir) or insulin glargine (Lantus), can be used to provide basal insulin because of its 24-hour duration of action, especially at night.

▶ If your pump used different basal rates throughout the day, choose a conservative dose for basal (long-acting) insulin injections. Use the lowest basal rate over a 24-hour period to calculate the amount of long-acting insulin to inject.

▶ Take into account the expected pump arrival time when deciding on the right time to take long-acting insulin. Meal and correction boluses using rapid-acting insulin will be required until you restart pump therapy.

there is no basal insulin. This can be a problem—who wants to stay up at night to give shots every four to six hours?

In most cases, long-acting insulin (insulin glargine [Lantus] or insulin detemir [Levemir]) is used to provide the basal insulin, and the rapid-acting insulin normally used in the pump is still used for meal and high blood glucose boluses. This regimen minimizes the need for frequent shots overnight. This method is helpful when you do not expect the replacement pump to arrive until the next day or later. However, it is important to remember that your specific needs for diabetes self-care may require different guidelines, so talk to your diabetes team before you begin taking insulin injections to make sure that this plan works best for you.

How Much Insulin?

During this period, your meal and high blood sugar doses will be the same as they were while you were on insulin pump therapy. This emphasizes why you need to have these doses written down beforehand, as described in the sidebar on page 47.

The hardest decision is figuring out *how much* long-acting insulin to use. One method is to add up all of the basal insulin provided each day and to give that as the long-acting insulin at bedtime or earlier, depending on when pump therapy was interrupted. You can calculate this manually, but pumps also provide that information in their settings. The problem with using the total basal rate is that the basal rate usually varies throughout the day. Using the total daily basal rate for your long-acting insulin dose does not take into account these changes. For example, if someone has a basal rate of 1 unit per hour from midnight to 6 A.M. and 1.5 units per hour the rest of the day, then the total basal insulin in a day is 33 units (6 hours at 1 unit per hour + 18 hours at 1.5 units per hour). In this example, the dose of insulin glargine (Lantus) or detemir (Levemir) might be 33 units, but that may be too much overnight (midnight to 6 A.M.) because the basal rate is much lower during that time than the rest of the day. Giving 33 units of long-acting insulin at bedtime may cause overnight hypoglycemia. It is therefore best to be conservative for the short time you will have to be on insulin injections. Use the lowest basal rate throughout the day to calculate the long-acting insulin dose. In the previous example, it is 1 unit per hour. This adds up to 24 units, so 24 units of long-acting insulin should be used.

Insulin glargine (Lantus) and insulin detemir (Levemir) do not have to be taken at night, but this tends to be a convenient time. When to take the dose may depend on when the pump is expected to arrive. Remember that these long-acting insulins work for up to 24 hours. So if your new pump arrives and is started while the long-acting insulin is still working, you may get too much insulin from the injection and the insulin pump. Prevent problems by writing down when you last injected long-acting insulin so you know when it will wear off. If your pump arrives early, wait for the long-acting insulin to wear off before restarting pump therapy. You will still be using rapid-acting insulin (for meals and high blood glucose levels) before and after long-acting insulin is taken.

As a reminder, contact your diabetes team for additional recommendations on how to handle insulin pump problems. Although many people who use insulin pumps will never have a problem with their pumps, planning for an emergency will guarantee that you are not caught unprepared.

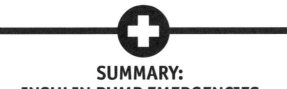

SUMMARY:
INSULIN PUMP EMERGENCIES

PUMP SUPPLY KIT INVENTORY

▶ Make two lists of all pump settings, including doses for meal boluses, high blood glucose boluses, and all basal rates and patterns. The lists should also include your target blood glucose levels, target ranges, etc. Some pump manufacturers allow you to download these settings to your home computer (or even to the manufacturer's online service over the Internet). This is a good way to keep a backup of your pump settings. Keep one list separate from the rest of your pump supply kit (in case you lose the pump supply kit).

▶ Be sure to have an adequate supply of rapid-acting insulin pens and pen needles available. If you use insulin syringes, be sure to have an adequate supply of them as well as insulin vials for day-to-day pump use.

▶ Keep some long-acting insulin pens or vials (e.g., insulin glargine [Lantus] or insulin detemir [Levemir]) available. The long-acting insulin may be used if injections are needed while waiting for a replacement pump.

▶ Keep extra pump batteries available at all times.

▶ Keep two or more extra infusion sets and related supplies.

CAUSES OF INTERRUPTED INSULIN DELIVERY

▶ empty reservoir (the pump is out of insulin)

▶ kinked tubing

▶ connection problems

▶ clogged or dislodged cannula

▶ leaking infusion set

▶ dead battery

▶ pump malfunction

Sometimes the cause of the problem is obvious, but other times some detective work is necessary.

GUIDELINES FOR PUMP PROBLEMS

When pump problems occur, follow these general guidelines.

▶ Check your blood glucose more often than usual, sometimes as often as every two hours.

▶ Check the pump, catheter tubing, and infusion site for obvious problems.

▶ If the cannula is out, insert a new infusion set and give a high blood glucose bolus using the pump and your usual correction dose.

▶ Check your urine for ketones when blood glucose levels are over 250 mg/dl. You will need more insulin if moderate or large amounts of urine ketones are present. Continue to check ketones. This can be useful in determining whether your situation is getting better or worse.

▶ Only give one high blood glucose bolus with the pump. If there is no response to that bolus (i.e., your blood glucose level has not changed or has increased) within two hours, an insulin injection needs to be given.

GUIDELINES FOR A TEMPORARY INSULIN REGIMEN

▶ Try contacting the pump manufacturer's local sales representative to get a replacement pump immediately rather than waiting for one to be shipped to you.

▶ *If you have a short wait for your replacement pump.* You can use rapid-acting insulin only (using your usual meal and correction bolus doses), but this requires injections every four to six hours. This is often not a problem during the day but can be inconvenient at night.

▶ *If you have a long wait for your replacement pump (24 hours or longer).* Long-acting insulin, such as insulin detemir (Levemir) or insulin glargine (Lantus), can be used to provide basal insulin because of its 24-hour duration of action, especially at night.

▶ If your pump used different basal rates throughout the day, choose a conservative dose for basal (long-acting) insulin injections. Use the lowest basal rate over a 24-hour period to calculate the amount of long-acting insulin to inject.

▶ Take into account the expected pump arrival time when deciding on the right time to take long-acting insulin. Meal and correction boluses using rapid-acting insulin will be required until you restart pump therapy.

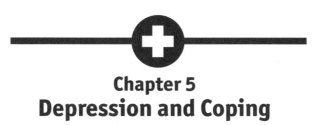

Chapter 5
Depression and Coping

Depression is common among children, adolescents, and adults with diabetes. One-third of people with diabetes experience depression at some point in their lives. Dealing with diabetes—as is the case with any chronic illness—takes strength and long-term survival skills. Diabetes is a high-maintenance process that has life-affecting consequences. Recognizing and dealing with short- and long-term frustrations are just as important as daily monitoring and medical treatment.

RECOGNIZING DEPRESSION

Depression is not always easy to recognize in yourself or others. Some of the signs of depression include: depressed mood, increased or decreased sleep, lack of interest in pleasurable activities, poor self-care, altered eating, feelings of hopelessness or helplessness, psychomotor agitation (unintentional and purposeless motions like pacing or fidgeting), psychomotor slowing (a state of under-

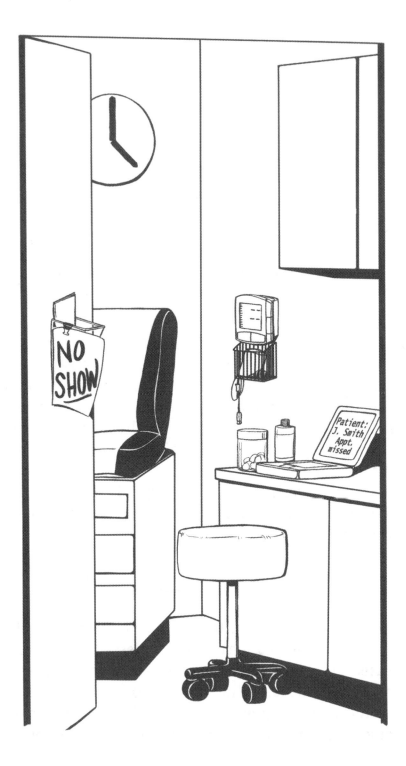

activity related to mental tension), and many others. The symptoms that indicate a person may have major depression are shown in the sidebar to the right.

If you suspect that you or a person with diabetes in your care may have depression, there are many screening questionnaires that look for depression. Contact your diabetes team for recommendations and referrals for help with depression. It is important to get help for depression because it can have a wide range of effects on a person, from mild to life-threatening consequences.

CRITERIA FOR MAJOR DEPRESSION

Major depression is likely if **five** of the following symptoms are present nearly every day for two weeks.

▶ Loss of interest and pleasure

▶ Change in sleep patterns

▶ Change in appetite and/or weight

▶ Low energy level/fatigue

▶ Psychomotor agitation/slowing

▶ Reduced ability to concentrate

▶ Low self-esteem or feelings of guilt

▶ Thoughts of suicide or death

Also, signs of depression in children and adolescents can include:

▶ Misbehavior, acting out

▶ Anger

▶ Social isolation

▶ Poor school performance

In Children and Teens

Children with diabetes can also experience depression. The symptoms of depression are similar in children and adolescents (see sidebar above), but can also include misbehavior, acting out, anger, social isolation, and poor school performance. Children do not typically recognize that they are depressed, so parents, teachers, sitters, and other caregivers have to be the ones who recognize changes in behavior.

Having diabetes during puberty can be very difficult. The teen-

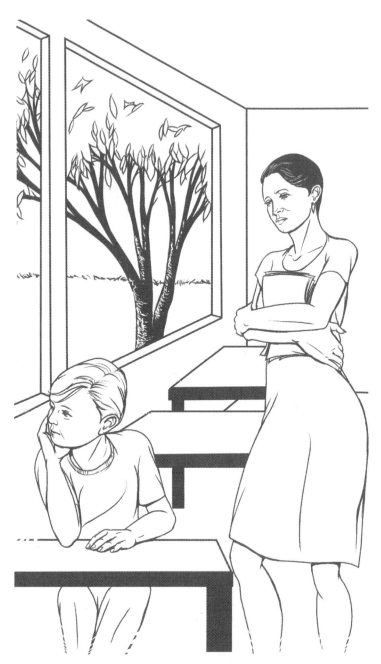

age years are a time when depression is already at higher risk, and the addition of diabetes raises that risk even more. Teenagers are often able to recognize the symptoms of depression in themselves, so teens may be able to seek help on their own. However, friends, family, and teachers are also good observers for changes in mood and other symptoms of depression and can help recognize and address depression in a teen.

In Adults

Being an adult does not protect you from the frustrations or depression that can accompany diabetes. Diabetes, like other chronic illnesses, can be involved in the development of depression. The more an illness affects daily activities, including the presence of complications, pain, and other chronic diseases (such as heart problems, high blood pressure, and vascular disorders), the more likely the person is to develop depression. Many studies have shown that people with diabetes (type 1 or type 2) and depression are more likely to develop diabetes complications, such as retinopathy, neuropathy, vascular disorders, and sexual dysfunction.

People with diabetes are twice as likely to experience depression at some point in their lives. Likewise, people with depression earlier in life are at higher risk of developing type 2 diabetes. Why this occurs is still unclear.

MEDICAL CONSEQUENCES OF DEPRESSION

Although probably not necessary, it is important to state the obvious: it is more difficult to take care of yourself if you are depressed! People with both diabetes and depression have more physical symptoms of diabetes (such as fatigue, increased urination, hunger, and shakiness), more days with symptoms, and more intense symptoms and are less likely to adjust properly to negative symptoms (like pain). Depression, when combined with diabetes, is a serious problem that needs to be treated.

How does depression affect blood glucose control? *In many ways.* Depression interferes with your ability to care for yourself. People who are depressed do not monitor their blood glucose levels as often as they should. Furthermore, people who are depressed are less likely to exercise; this can lead to even higher glucose levels and weight gain. Lastly, people with depression tend to eat more and eat higher-calorie items, both of which lead to higher blood glucose.

Many people with depression use food as a coping mechanism. Obviously, this can be a problem for people who also have diabetes. Comfort foods tend to have more calories and carbohydrates, leading to higher blood glucose levels and weight gain. For other people, depression leads to eating less and, in some cases, avoiding food altogether. Not eating food increases the risks for hypoglycemia and malnutrition. Sometimes, the decision to eat more or less can be a sign of new or reemerging eating disorders, such as anorexia nervosa and bulimia. These are serious, potentially life-threatening illnesses that need to be appropriately treated by doctors specializing in these conditions.

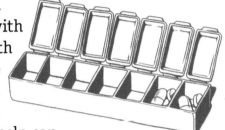

Depression can also interfere with receiving appropriate care. People with depression tend to have a harder time taking their medications, which can lead to higher blood glucose levels. Just getting to the people who can help can be hard, too. People with depression are more likely to miss appointments with their health care providers, including primary care physicians, diabetes specialists, educators, eye doctors, dentists, and mental health providers.

Drinking alcohol or drug abuse can also be a coping mechanism for depression. Alcohol affects the body's glucose production and glucose regulation, and it adds calories. High levels of alcohol consumption radically increase the risk of hypoglycemia (see page 22). Chronic alcohol use is a dangerous illness that requires care.

Having a Child with Diabetes

Raising a child can be challenging in and of itself. However, the parents of a child with diabetes have many more issues with which to cope, in addition to the usual stresses of childrearing. Parents of a child with diabetes can go through a range of emotions, including anger, frustration, and guilt. These can be overwhelming at times and may lead to depression. Parental depression will certainly affect a child's diabetes management, so seeking help is critical for the well-being of both parents and their children. Many parent support groups deal with this aspect particularly well.

WHAT RESOURCES ARE AVAILABLE?

There are many resources available to provide help if you have depression, some formal and some informal. Sometimes it is best to seek professional help from a psychiatrist, psychologist, or social worker. Medications are available for the treatment of depression. Newer medications are safe and effective and are less likely to have side effects.

Counseling and support are offered by many community centers, hospitals, youth groups, and religious organizations. Being part of a support group is usually helpful for everyone involved. Sometimes you will be the person providing support, sometimes you will be receiving support, and other times, there will be a mixture of both.

TREATMENT OPTIONS FOR PEOPLE WITH DEPRESSION

▶ Antidepressant medications

▶ Psychotherapy (for all forms of depression)

▶ Psychosocial interventions

▶ Support groups

Being a role model to others is a vital responsibility and often greatly underestimated.

A perfect example of the importance of being a role model was witnessed on a recent airline flight. Two strangers sitting next to each other were getting ready to eat the snack purchased on board. One took out a blood glucose meter and checked her glucose. Seeing this, the other passenger said that she also had diabetes but would never check her blood glucose in public. After checking her glucose, the first passenger asked the flight attendant how many carbohydrates were in the different snacks. The flight attendant did not know immediately but knew where to find the information and offered to look it up for her. When the flight attendant returned, the three of them had a conversation about diabetes. All of them had diabetes, so they discussed how they dealt with time changes during travel, airplane food, and coping with security. It was a useful interaction for all. This example shows how support can arrive in your life at any time, and it never would have happened if that first passenger had not checked her blood glucose right there on the plane.

Remember, it is very important to deal with depression. It has widespread effects on health. So, look for depression and, if it is there, address it!

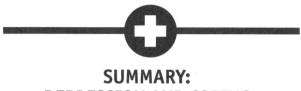

SUMMARY:
DEPRESSION AND COPING

CRITERIA FOR MAJOR DEPRESSION

Major depression is likely if **five** of the following symptoms are present nearly every day for two weeks.

▶ Loss of interest and pleasure

▶ Change in sleep patterns

▶ Change in appetite and/or weight

▶ Low energy level/fatigue

▶ Psychomotor agitation/slowing

▶ Reduced ability to concentrate

▶ Low self-esteem or feelings of guilt

▶ Thoughts of suicide or death

Also, signs of depression in children/adolescents can include misbehavior, acting out, anger, social isolation, or poor school performance.

RESOURCES FOR HELP WITH DEPRESSION

▶ Psychiatrists

▶ Psychologists

▶ School counselors

▶ Social workers

▶ Religious support groups

▶ Community support groups

▶ Camps

▶ Friends and family

▶ Other people with diabetes

TREATMENT OPTIONS FOR PEOPLE WITH DEPRESSION

▶ Antidepressant medications

▶ Psychotherapy (for all forms of depression)

▶ Psychosocial interventions

▶ Support groups

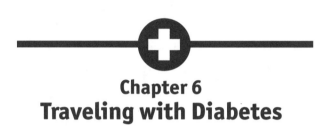

Chapter 6
Traveling with Diabetes

Traveling can be a challenge for anyone, but for those with diabetes it can be even more difficult because of the many medications and supplies they must carry with them at all times. In this chapter, we cover many issues that arise during travel, including dealing with airport security, getting prescriptions and supplies when overseas, some domestic travel problems (such as leaving everything at the hotel), insulin management when overseas, and crossing time zones.

LEAVING HOME

Like the other topics we've covered, *prevention* is the key to avoiding problems when traveling. One way to do this is to create a checklist of things you will need during your trip. Review your checklist while packing so you do not forget anything important. Even things you think you would never forget, like your insulin pump, could be left behind when you're excited about a trip or in a hurry to catch a

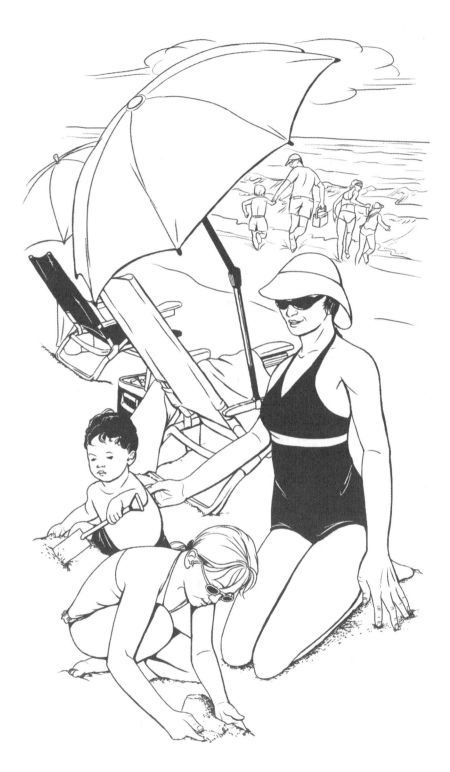

flight. A helpful checklist is provided in the sidebar below. Having the diabetes supply kit discussed in chapter 1 will be helpful, too, and it includes most of the items in this checklist.

Packing wisely will help reduce the chance of problems later on. Keep all of your supplies and insulin in your carry-on luggage. There are two reasons for this. First, you don't want to be without your supplies if your luggage is lost. Second, checked baggage is subjected to extreme temperatures that may badly affect insulin and other supplies. If you cannot take everything in your carry-on luggage (for example, if you will be gone for several weeks), carry on at least half of your supplies (but all of your insulin) and put the remaining supplies in your checked luggage. Pack insulin between clothing or something soft so insulin vials will not break. Do not

TRAVELER'S CHECKLIST

▶ Insulin pump (plus an extra one in case there are problems)
▶ Insulin pump supplies: plenty of infusion sets, reservoirs, batteries, and transparent dressings (if you use them)
▶ List of insulin pump settings, including basal rates, meal boluses, and high blood glucose target and sensitivity settings
▶ Diabetes medicines (insulin and diabetes pills) and extra (in case you lose some)
▶ Blood glucose test strips
▶ Lancets
▶ Alcohol wipes
▶ Urine ketone strips (and blood ketone test strips, if used)
▶ Items to treat mild or moderate low blood glucose levels, such as juice boxes, glucose tablets, etc.
▶ Glucagon emergency kits (bring at least two)
▶ Insulin syringes and/or pen needles
▶ Blood glucose meters (bring two) and extra batteries
▶ Prescriptions for medicines and insulin
▶ Letter from your doctor

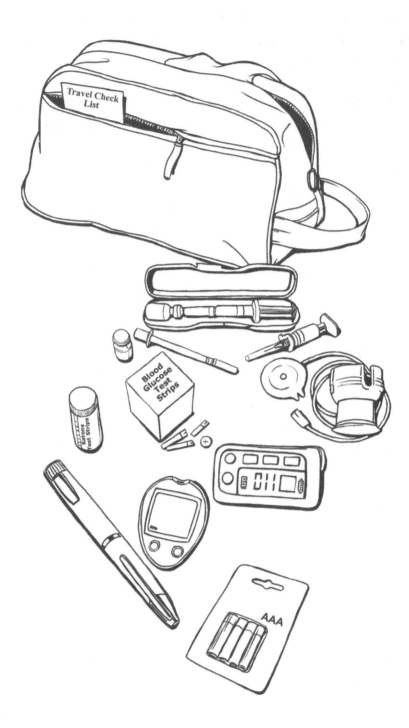

place insulin pumps, even backups, in your checked luggage. You would hate to lose your pump for two reasons: they are very expensive to replace and you may need it. When packing, be prepared for lost luggage.

Did you know that most, if not all, pump companies will provide an extra "vacation" insulin pump for while you are traveling? This can be helpful if your insulin pump breaks and you will not be able to get a replacement during your travels. Talk to your pump company about this well in advance of your trip. Bear in mind that you may be charged for this service and will have to return the extra pump to the company when you get back from vacation.

If you are on an insulin pump, take a bottle or two of long-acting (insulin glargine [Lantus] or insulin detemir [Levemir]) and short-acting insulins, along with syringes or insulin pens in case you have to use injections. In general, the amount of long-acting insulin you will need would be the minimum amount of basal insulin you get in a day (see chapter 4). Your meal bolus and high blood glucose bolus doses will be the same as if you were still on the pump.

Last, take plenty of extra supplies. Bring twice the amount you think you will need while you are away. This includes all blood glucose testing supplies (lancets, strips, an extra blood glucose meter, batteries, etc.), urine and/or ketone strips, glucagon (at least two kits), insulin, other medications, syringes, pump supplies, and basically everything listed in the checklist on page 71. Take at least one more bottle of each type of insulin than you think you will need.

BEFORE YOU FLY

Flight delays, crowded airports, long lines...these are all common barriers to a stress-free trip. You can do a few things before you fly to make the trip a little—or a lot—better.

▶ Call the airline 24 hours in advance to confirm your flight. If

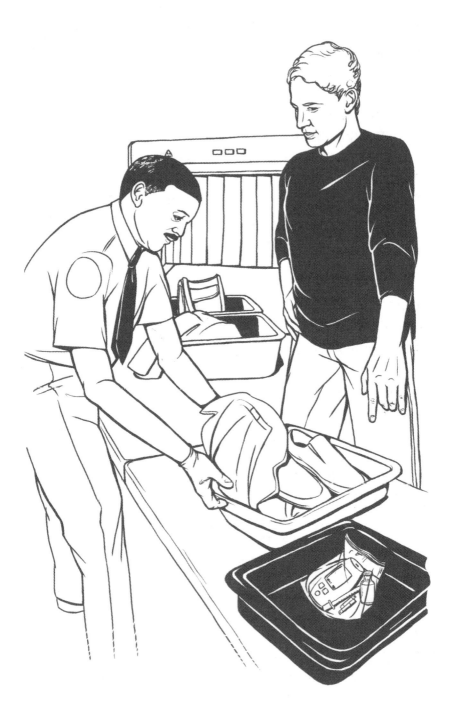

you don't, you run the risk of getting bumped if the flight is overbooked. Just having assigned seats does not guarantee that you have a seat on the flight if you do not confirm your flight in advance.

▶ Use online check-in whenever possible. Doing this helps eliminate some of the long lines at the airport. It will also confirm your flight. Many, if not all, airlines allow you to check in online, even if you have to check luggage.

▶ Remember that most airlines do not offer meals for domestic travel unless you are flying a great distance. Call the airlines ahead of time or check online flight information to determine whether meals are provided or available. If not, bring snacks or a meal on board.

▶ If a meal is provided, call the airline a few days in advance to request a special meal, such as a low-fat or low-cholesterol meal, and get carbohydrate content information. A low-carbohydrate meal is not always necessary, depending on the treatment regimen used, but is recommended as well. Always take along extra snacks because of possible delays.

AIRPORT SECURITY

Going through airport security can be a hassle even for people who don't have diabetes. Long lines and making sure you don't have items that will be confiscated make every trip through airline security a challenge. The latest rules from the U.S. Transportation Security Authority (TSA) limit the amount of fluids taken on board a plane. However, insulin and other medicines are excluded from this limitation and do not count toward the one-quart bag limit of three-ounce fluid containers. In fact, all diabetes supplies are allowed through the checkpoint after they are screened by security. The TSA website (www.tsa.dhs.gov) has information about traveling with diabetes. It is advisable that you visit this web-

Tips for a Hassle-Free
Trip Through Airport Security

▶ Notify the security officer that you have diabetes and have diabetes supplies in your bag.

▶ All medications (including insulin vials, insulin pens, and glucagon kits) should be clearly labeled with the name of the patient (pharmacy label should be intact).

▶ Keep the boxes for your insulin vials (don't tear off the pharmacy labels).

▶ Items for treating hypoglycemia, such as juice boxes, are allowed and should be exempt from the one-quart bag limitation. If you're concerned about losing them, pack other treatment forms, such as glucose tablets.

▶ If you have an insulin pump, notify the security officer before going through the metal detector so a visual inspection of the pump can be performed.

▶ Lancets can be brought on board if they are accompanied by a blood glucose meter.

▶ Blood glucose meters should have the manufacturer's name imprinted on the meter.

▶ Carry a letter from your diabetes center that states that you have diabetes and need to take diabetes supplies with you.

▶ Carry a copy of all of your written prescriptions.

site each and every time you fly because procedures continue to change; just search at the top right portion of the TSA home page for "diabetes."

Nothing on the TSA website indicates that you need to have a letter from your physician or copies of prescriptions. However, some airlines have indicated that passengers need such a letter, and it is a good idea to have copies of prescriptions whenever you travel just in case you need an emergency refill. Be safe; get a letter from your diabetes center and carry copies of your prescriptions when you travel. A sample letter is on page 77.

This is a sample letter from your diabetes center that should accompany you or your child when traveling. It should be printed on your diabetes center's official letterhead. For children, use your child's name and make other changes as needed.

[Diabetes Center Name]
[Diabetes Center Street Address]
[Diabetes Center City, State, and ZIP Code]
[Diabetes Center Phone Number]

RE: [your name and date of birth]

To Whom It May Concern:

[Your name] has type 1 [or type 2] diabetes and is currently under my care at [Diabetes Center Name]. For Mr./Mrs./Ms. [your last name] to properly care for his [or her] diabetes while traveling, he [or she] will need to carry diabetes care items with them on the plane.

It is necessary for Mr./Mrs./Ms. [your last name] to have immediate access to his [or her] blood glucose meter, insulin syringes/vials or insulin pens, lancets, lancet device, glucagon emergency kit, ketone test strips, skin care items, dressing material, glucose tablets or gel, and any food items to manage low blood glucose levels. These items need to be kept out of extreme heat and cold. Mr./Mrs./Ms. [your last name] should not be detained during meal or snack times because of the possibility of a low blood glucose reaction, which could become life threatening.

Thank you for your cooperation in this matter. Please do not hesitate to contact me if you have any questions.

Sincerely,

[Doctor's name and title]

AVOIDING COMMON PROBLEMS

Most problems while traveling are just a slight bump in your plans. You can avoid most of these common problems. Once you have arrived at your destination, what can you do to keep your diabetes care uninterrupted?

A common problem is running out of insulin, other medicines, or other diabetes supplies. This may happen for many reasons: lost luggage, broken insulin vials, or supplies left behind in a hotel or taxi are just a few. Although we cannot always prevent such mistakes, we can take measures to help prevent little mistakes from turning into potentially dangerous disasters (see sidebar on page 78).

TIPS TO AVOID PROBLEMS WHILE TRAVELING

▶ Check your blood glucose frequently while traveling, including before and two to three hours after meals. You may be eating unfamiliar foods that have unknown effects on your blood glucose levels. Checking your blood glucose levels after eating is the best way to assess the different effects different foods have on you. Plus, the excitement of being on vacation or in a new place may also affect your blood glucose levels.

▶ Perform frequent control tests on your meter with the control solution, especially when traveling in warm, humid climates. Heat and humidity can affect glucose meters and test strips.

▶ Pay attention to your activity level. Some vacations are relaxed, whereas others are more active and you're always on the go. Your insulin needs may increase or decrease, depending on how active you are.

▶ Carry copies of all of your prescriptions with you. Many nationwide pharmacy chains are electronically linked by their computer networks. If you are out of town and happen to be in a city with one of those chain pharmacies and need supplies, you can go to that pharmacy for refills.

▶ Be sure your insulin is not exposed to extreme temperatures, especially excess heat. Just like at home, keep your insulin as well as your meter and test strips out of direct sunlight when traveling. Using a small cooler when you are in sunny areas, such as theme parks, water parks, and the beach, can help keep the insulin from going bad. Also remember that while outdoors, insulin in a bag or backpack may overheat.

▶ Be sure insulin is safely packed to prevent breakage.

▶ Always carry items you use to treat hypoglycemia, such as glucose tablets or juice boxes.

▶ Don't forget to take glucagon with you, and be sure your travel companions know how to use it.

▶ Make dining reservations whenever possible. This helps avoid long delays.

▶ Carry snacks at all times in case of unexpected delays. Do not assume that you will be able to find food everywhere you go.

▶ Pack extra water. Water, especially when you are outside in the heat, can be a lifesaver.

TRAVELING ABROAD

Although you don't have to travel overseas to run into problems with diabetes, being in another country can make a bad problem

---

TIPS FOR TRAVELING ABROAD

▶ Obtain the name of English-speaking physicians practicing in foreign countries before you travel. The International Association for Medical Assistance to Travellers (www.iamat.org) can provide a list of English-speaking physicians in foreign countries. The International Diabetes Federation (www.idf.org) may be able to help you find approved diabetes organizations and groups overseas. You might also want to contact the local U.S. embassy as well.

▶ Keep a small phrase book handy at all times.

▶ Learn some common diabetes phrases that may be required in case of emergency. Here are a few important phrases that you should know in the local language: "I have diabetes," "Please call an ambulance," "I need a pharmacy," and "Some juice or sugar, please."

▶ If you need to obtain a vial of insulin while traveling in a foreign country, keep in mind that the insulin may not be in the same concentration as what you normally use. Almost all insulin in the U.S. is U-100 concentration, meaning there are 100 units of insulin per milliliter volume. Some countries use U-40 or U-80 concentrations (only 40 or 80 units of insulin per milliliter, respectively). If you use your own syringes, which are meant for U-100 insulin, with other concentrations, you will not be getting the right amount of insulin. You will also need to purchase syringes that match the insulin concentration. Be sure that you use the correct syringe with the proper insulin concentrations.

▶ If you obtain a vial of insulin while abroad, stick with the same brand and formulation as you use at home. If your brand is not available, you can substitute another manufacturer's equivalent brand (for example, NovoLog for Humalog, Humulin R for Novolin R). Keep in mind that name brands differ, so look at the generic name to be sure you are getting the same insulin (i.e., NovoLog is insulin aspart, Humalog is insulin lispro).

worse. Language barriers, different social customs (for example, timing of meals), being in unfamiliar territory, and other reasons contribute to the problems you may face when traveling abroad.

Follow the recommendations in the sidebar on page 79 to minimize the chances that you will have problems when traveling overseas.

CROSSING TIME ZONES

A difficult task that accompanies traveling is learning how to adjust insulin doses when crossing time zones. How do you deal with jet lag? How do you address the fact that your meal times are different from normal? These questions may surface whenever you travel. The best first step is to visit your doctor a few weeks before leaving—or to call your diabetes center—so you can have these questions answered. This will give everyone a chance to review your itinerary and make recommendations for your insulin regimen.

TACKLING TIME ZONES

Many different insulin regimens are available today, so we will not offer any specific recommendations. Here are basic guidelines for traveling across time zones—but remember to discuss your needs with your diabetes team well in advance.

▶ In general, crossing fewer than four or five time zones will not require a major change in your insulin regimen. If you are flying eastward (e.g., U.S. to Europe), the day of flight will be shorter and you may require less insulin. This is because insulin doses will be given closer to each other than normal. If you are flying westward (e.g., Europe to the U.S.), the day of flight will be longer and you may need more insulin. Depending on flight time and duration, delays, and other factors, you may not need to make changes to your insulin regimen.

▶ If you use an insulin pump, managing time zone changes is much easier. The bolus doses (for both meal and high blood glucose) will not change. You may have to change your basal rate to match the new time zone in which you are located.

▶ If you are not already on a basal-bolus insulin injection regimen (insulin glargine [Lantus] or insulin detemir [Levemir] for basal needs, plus a rapid-acting insulin for meal and high blood glucose boluses), changing to this mode of therapy may make the trip a lot easier. This is the best way to mimic your own body's insulin production, short of using an insulin pump. Talk to your diabetes team about switching to this insulin regimen for your trip. You may even want to stay on this therapy afterward because of the flexibility it provides.

▶ Be sure to check your blood glucose levels frequently while flying, at least once every four hours.

▶ Keep yourself well hydrated while flying. Drink plenty of water or other nonalcoholic, caffeine-free, and sugar-free beverages.

▶ Do not set your watch to the new time zone until you arrive at your destination. It will be easier to figure out when you'll need more insulin.

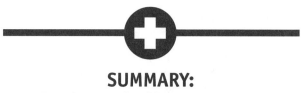

SUMMARY:
TRAVELING WITH DIABETES

TRAVELER'S CHECKLIST

- Insulin pump (plus an extra one in case there are problems)
- Insulin pump supplies: plenty of infusion sets, reservoirs, batteries, and transparent dressings (if you use them)
- List of insulin pump settings, including basal rates, meal boluses, and high blood glucose target and sensitivity settings
- Diabetes medicines (insulin and diabetes pills) and extra (in case you lose some)
- Blood glucose test strips
- Lancets
- Alcohol wipes
- Urine ketone strips (and blood ketone test strips, if used)
- Items to treat mild or moderate low blood glucose levels, such as juice boxes, glucose tablets, etc.
- Glucagon emergency kits (bring at least two)
- Insulin syringes and/or pen needles
- Blood glucose meters (bring two) and extra batteries
- Prescriptions for medicines and insulin
- Letter from your doctor

BEFORE YOU FLY

You can do a few things before you fly to make the trip a little—or a lot—better.

- Call the airline 24 hours in advance to confirm your flight. If you don't, you run the risk of getting bumped if the flight is overbooked. Just having assigned seats does not guarantee that you have a seat on the flight if you do not confirm your flight in advance.

- Use online check-in whenever possible. Doing this helps eliminate some of the long lines at the airport. It will also confirm your flight. Many, if not all, airlines allow you to check in online, even if you have to check luggage.

- Remember that most airlines do not offer meals for domestic travel unless you are flying a great distance. Call the airlines ahead of time or check online flight information to determine whether meals are provided. If not, bring snacks or a meal on board.

- If a meal is provided, call the airline a few days in advance to request a special meal, such as a low-fat or low-cholesterol meal, and get carbohydrate content information. A low-carbohydrate meal is not always necessary, depending on the treatment regimen used, but is recommended as well. Always take along extra snacks because of possible delays.

TIPS FOR A HASSLE-FREE TRIP THROUGH AIRPORT SECURITY

- Notify the security officer that you have diabetes and have diabetes supplies in your bag.

- All medications (including insulin vials, insulin pens, and glucagon kits) should be clearly labeled with the name of the patient (pharmacy label should be intact).

- Keep the boxes for your insulin vials (don't tear off the pharmacy labels).

- Items for treating hypoglycemia, such as juice boxes, are allowed and should be exempt from the one-quart bag limitation. If you're concerned about losing them, pack other treatment forms, such as glucose tablets.

- If you have an insulin pump, notify the security officer before going through the metal detector so a visual inspection of the pump can be performed.

- Lancets can be brought on board if they are accompanied by a blood glucose meter.

- Blood glucose meters should have the manufacturer's name imprinted on the meter.

- Carry a letter from your diabetes center that states that you have diabetes and need to take diabetes supplies with you.
- Carry a copy of all of your written prescriptions.

TIPS TO AVOID PROBLEMS WHILE TRAVELING

- Check your blood glucose frequently while traveling, including before and two to three hours after meals.
- Perform frequent control tests on your meter with the control solution, especially when traveling in warm, humid climates.
- Pay attention to your activity level. Some vacations are relaxed, whereas others are more active and you're always on the go. Your insulin needs may increase or decrease, depending on how active you are.
- Carry copies of all of your prescriptions with you. Using one of the chain pharmacies can help get easy prescription refills during domestic travel.
- Be sure your insulin is not exposed to extreme temperatures, especially excess heat. Use a small cooler when you are outside in the sun to help keep insulin from going bad. Also remember that while outdoors, insulin kept in a bag or backpack may overheat.
- Be sure insulin is safely packed to prevent breakage.
- Always carry items you use to treat hypoglycemia, such as glucose tablets or juice boxes.
- Don't forget to take glucagon with you, and be sure your travel companions know how to use it.
- Make dining reservations whenever possible. This helps avoid long delays.
- Carry snacks at all times in case of unexpected delays. Do not assume that you will be able to find food everywhere you go.
- Pack extra water. Water, especially when you are outside in the heat, can be a lifesaver.

TIPS FOR TRAVELING ABROAD

- Obtain the name of English-speaking physicians practicing in foreign countries before you travel. The International Association for Medical Assistance to Travellers (www.iamat.org) can provide a list of English-speaking physicians in foreign countries. The International Diabetes Federation (www.idf.org) may be able to help you find approved diabetes organizations and groups overseas. You might also want to contact the local U.S. embassy as well.

- Keep a small phrase book handy at all times.

- Learn some common diabetes phrases that may be required in case of emergency. Here are a few important phrases that you should know in the local language: "I have diabetes," "Please call an ambulance," "I need a pharmacy," and "Some juice or sugar, please."

- If you need to obtain a vial of insulin while traveling in a foreign country, be sure to check the insulin's concentration (e.g., U-40 or U-80). You will also need to purchase syringes that match the insulin concentration.

- If you obtain a vial of insulin while abroad, stick with the same brand and formulation as you use at home. If your brand is not available, substitute another manufacturer's equivalent brand (for example, NovoLog for Humalog, Humulin R for Novolin R). Name brands differ, so look at the generic name to be sure you are getting the same insulin (i.e., NovoLog is insulin aspart, Humalog is insulin lispro).

TACKLING TIME ZONES

Here are a few basic guidelines for traveling across time zones, but remember to discuss your needs with your diabetes team beforehand.

- In general, crossing fewer than four or five time zones will not require a major change in your insulin regimen. If you are flying eastward (e.g., U.S. to Europe), the day of flight will be shorter and you may require less insulin. If you are flying westward (e.g., Europe to the U.S.), the day of flight will be longer and you may need more insulin. Depending on flight time and duration, delays, and other factors, you may not need to make changes to your insulin regimen.

▶ If you use an insulin pump, managing time zone changes is much easier. The bolus doses (for both meal and high blood glucose) will not change. You may have to change your basal rate to match the time zone in which you are located.

▶ If you are not already on a basal-bolus insulin injection regimen (insulin glargine [Lantus] or insulin detemir [Levemir] for basal needs, plus a rapid-acting insulin for meal and high blood glucose boluses), changing to this mode of therapy may make the trip a lot easier. This is the best way to mimic your own body's insulin production, short of using an insulin pump. Talk to your diabetes team about switching to this insulin regimen for your trip. You may even want to stay on this therapy afterward because of the flexibility it provides.

▶ Be sure to check your blood glucose levels frequently while flying, at least once every four hours.

▶ Keep yourself well hydrated while flying. Drink plenty of water or other nonalcoholic, caffeine-free, and sugar-free beverages.

▶ Do not set your watch to the new time zone until you arrive at your destination. It will be easier to figure out when you'll need more insulin.

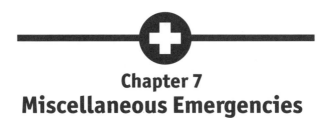

Chapter 7
Miscellaneous Emergencies

There are many diabetes-related problems that may not be "true" emergencies, but they are still important and demand attention. Most of these emergencies are more important for adults with diabetes. Be sure to talk to your diabetes team about which problems can occur in children.

EYE EMERGENCIES

Many people with diabetes are afraid of losing their vision. It is important to have your eyes regularly evaluated, which can help prevent many long-term problems. An eye evaluation may include a dilated eye exam (to examine the sensing layer of the eye, or retina, and its nerves and blood vessels), special tests to look for fluid under the retina, and pressure tests (to make sure the eye is not under too much pressure, which may lead to a condition called *glaucoma*). An eye doctor will also check to see if you have or are at risk for *diabetic retinopathy*, a serious condition in which long-term high blood glucose levels damage the blood ves-

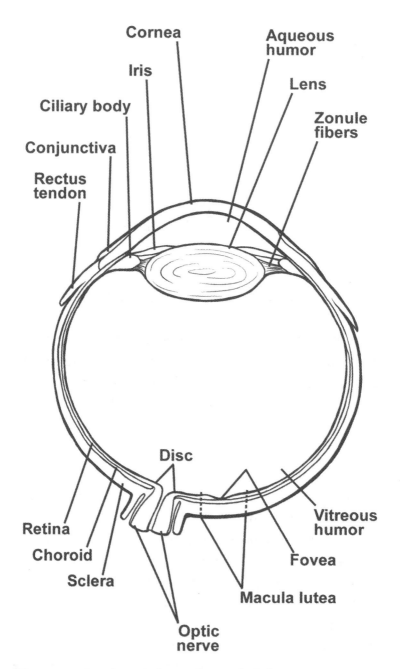

Cornea

Aqueous
humor

Iris

Lens

Ciliary body

Zonule
fibers

Conjunctiva

Rectus
tendon

Disc

Retina

Vitreous
humor

Choroid

Fovea

Sclera

Macula lutea

Optic
nerve

Diagram, horizontal section of right eye

sels and nerves in the eye, leading to loss of vision. Having your eyes checked on a regular basis can catch and usually prevent eye problems. *Remember, most vision loss is preventable!*

The eye has several different areas that need to function properly for you to see. These include (but are not limited to) the cornea, lens, retina, and optic nerve (a long nerve that travels to the part of the brain that organizes the information from the eye). Problems that need immediate attention can occur at several places. The outer layer (or cornea)—the part of your eye that you see in the mirror—may become infected. Some cornea infections just require time to heal; others will require antibiotics or anti-inflammatory drugs. It is hard to tell whether you have a viral conjunctivitis like pink eye or a life-threatening infection by just looking in the mirror. It is important to see your eye doctor immediately so treatment, if needed, can begin right away.

The lens, the part of the eye that focuses light, can become cloudy over time. When the clouding increases enough to obstruct vision, it is called a *cataract*. Cataracts develop in everyone as they age, but people with diabetes tend to develop them earlier. In some cases, this can occur very rapidly, over just days or weeks. If this happens, your ability to see will degrade rapidly.

The most frightening eye problems are the ones that occur rapidly or are present when you wake up. The two most common causes of these severe problems are bleeding into the vitreous (the fluid-filled center of the eye) and detachment of the retina. These are both serious emergencies. If blood gets into the vitreous, it becomes cloudy and light cannot pass through it to the retina, which reduces vision. This is usually caused by leaking blood vessels in the retina, which in turn is often caused by diabetic retinopathy. Detachment of the retina is also very serious. A detached retina can no longer detect light and thus causes blurred vision and may lead to complete blindness. Because these eye problems are quite serious, an abrupt loss in vision or flashing or floating lights should be taken very seriously. You need to contact your eye doctor immediately or head to the emergency room if these symptoms are present.

Other Eye Emergencies

Cranial nerve palsies can arise in many different forms because there are several nerves that can be affected by this disorder (*palsy* means that a nerve is not working properly). The most common nerve affected by cranial nerve palsy is the nerve that controls the upper eyelid and allows you to lift it and open your eye. If this nerve is affected, you will not be able to see because you cannot open your upper eyelid. It is very frightening to awaken and not be able to see. This is usually a result of nerve damage from lack of blood supply and/or high blood glucose. Other nerves can be affected, including the ones that control which way the eye turns (your eyes go in different directions). This can give you double vision.

Glaucoma is a disease that damages the optic nerve, which is the nerve that transmits vision information to the brain and allows us to see. An increase of pressure inside the eye can lead to glaucoma, but that is not the only known cause of this disease. There are many areas in the eye that need to be regularly checked for glaucoma. Untreated glaucoma can lead to mild to moderate loss of vision and even blindness in more serious cases. Usually, glaucoma has no noticeable symptoms, but severe or rapidly progressing glaucoma can cause eye pain and/or redness.

SIGNS OF AN EYE EMERGENCY

▶ Loss of vision

▶ Eye pain

▶ Double or blurred vision

▶ Redness of the eye

▶ Floating or flashing lights

FOOT EMERGENCIES

Many people with diabetes worry about losing a limb, particularly their feet. This diabetes problem can be prevented with proper care and a careful eye. There are two key goals in keeping your feet safe and healthy. First, you need to prevent nerve and vessel damage in your feet (and other limbs). You can achieve this by maintaining healthy blood glucose levels and working to keep them in the target range. Second, you need to *protect your feet*. Don't put them in harm's way. You can do this by wearing good, thick socks and properly fitting shoes all the time, both outdoors and inside. Cotton, dye-free socks designed specifically for people with diabetes are available, as are form-fitted shoes and inserts. You will also need to inspect and clean your feet every day.

If the nerves in your feet become damaged, you may not feel a blister forming, a rock caught in your shoe, or even if you have stepped on a nail! Inspect your feet every day. If you find an ulcer or infection, see your doctor immediately. Make it a goal to maintain excellent foot and nail care, too, especially if the shape of your foot changes (for example, if you have bunions, hammer toes, or fallen arches). If your foot sensation is not normal because of diabetic nerve damage, small fractures in the feet that go untreated can lead to extreme changes in foot shape. The foot can become red and hot when this happens. Avoid this dangerous complication by taking the time to inspect and care for your feet daily. Have your diabetes team demonstrate how to properly inspect your feet every day.

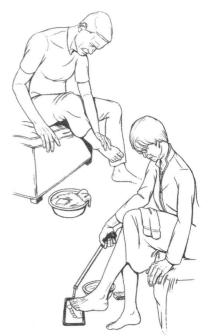

Loss of Blood to the Feet

Be sure that you are always receiving enough blood to your feet. If you are not, this can turn into a very serious emergency! Reduced blood flow to the foot can be caused by narrowed arteries to the leg, blood clots in these arteries, or clots traveling from other parts of the body and lodging in these arteries. If you are not receiving enough blood in any limb, then it is at risk of being amputated, so seek help quickly. Loss of blood supply does not happen frequently, but if it does, time is of the essence. Reestablishing blood flow needs to be done as soon as possible! The signs of this condition are usually obvious, even if you do not have perfect sensation, and should not be ignored.

SIGNS OF LOSS OF BLOOD TO THE FEET

▶ Pain

▶ Cool to the touch, lack of warmth

▶ Pale skin, lack of color

▶ No pulse

CARDIOVASCULAR EMERGENCIES

Heart disease is very common in adults with diabetes, as well as in those with pre-diabetes and insulin resistance. The two most common emergencies are probably familiar to you; they are heart attacks and strokes.

Heart Attack

In most cases, the warning sign of a heart attack is a mid-chest crushing pressure; some people describe it as feeling like an elephant is sitting on their chest. This can be accompanied by several other symptoms, including shortness of breath, nausea, or arm or jaw pain. Symptoms are usually worsened by activity and improved with rest. If you have diabetic neuropathy (nerve damage caused by high blood glucose levels), you may not easily recognize the signs of a heart attack. Some other signs of a heart attack can include pain in the back or neck. Note that these other signs are a little more common in women experiencing a heart attack.

If you suspect you are having a heart attack, seek help immediately. Call 911. The faster you are evaluated and treated, the better the outcome! If you think you may be having a heart attack, it is not safe to drive yourself.

Stroke

A stroke is a very dangerous condition caused by reduced blood flow to the brain. Because a stroke affects different parts of the brain, there can be many different symptoms (see sidebar on page 94). You can have difficulty seeing, numbness or weakness, loss of balance or muscle control, or any combination of these.

You can prevent a stroke by working toward your target levels in blood glucose, lipids (cholesterol and triglycerides), and blood pressure. Because strokes are often caused by blood clots, daily use of aspirin may be helpful in adults. Many adults with diabetes are instructed to take a "baby" dose aspirin (81 mg) once a day. However, this is not good for all people with diabetes, so discuss with your diabetes team whether you should be taking aspirin daily.

Sometimes, the results of a stroke are temporary or can be reversed with medicines. The key factor in recovering from a stroke is *time*—how long it takes to get treatment. As with heart attacks, the faster you are evaluated and treated, the better the outcome! If you have any reason to you think you are having a stroke, *immediately* call 911 or have someone take you to the nearest emergency room. *Do not wait.*

SIGNS OF A STROKE

▶ Sudden numbness or weakness in the face, arm, or leg

▶ Confusion

▶ Difficulty speaking or understanding

▶ Trouble seeing

▶ Loss of balance or muscle control

▶ Sudden, severe headache

MEDICAL ALERT IDENTIFICATION

Having medical alert identification is one thing you hope to never need, but having it can save your life. If you are in a situation in which you cannot communicate that you have diabetes, it is important that others can find out that you have diabetes or other medical conditions. Medical alert identification is most often carried in the wallet (next to the driver's license or ID card) or on the body in a recognizable area (for example, a bracelet or necklace). If someone is having a medical emergency, police, emergency medical technicians, and public awareness trainees are often taught to look for medical information in these places. If you place a card in your wallet, make sure it contains the following information: it states that you have diabetes, what medicines you are taking, and

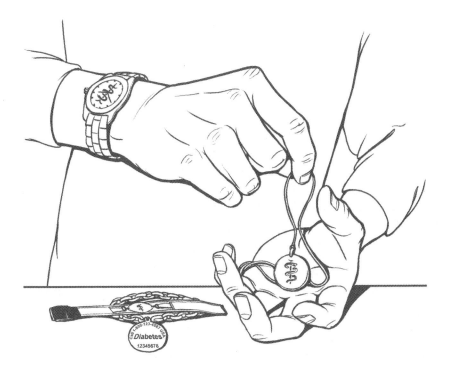

what to do if you cannot help yourself (for example, "If I am unconscious, I may be having a low blood sugar reaction.").

There are many jewelry-like items, such as necklaces, bracelets, and watches, which can be engraved with a medical alert symbol and the word "diabetes." Name and emergency contact information are also often engraved on these items. Emergency personnel are trained to look for medical alert identifications around the neck

SOME MEDICAL ALERT IDENTIFICATION COMPANIES

▶ American Medical ID: www.americanmedical-id.com

▶ Medic Alert: www.medicalert.org

▶ Medic I.D.: www.medic-id.com

▶ Medic ID'S International: www.medicid.com

▶ MedIDs.com: www.medids.com

▶ Vital-ID: www.medicalwristband.com

and the wrists, so make the information easy to find and keep the identification item in one of those places. Medical alert identification is made by many companies and is easily purchased (see sidebar on page 95). They can be as simple or elaborate as you want, but be sure that they are clearly medical identifications and will not be mistaken for regular jewelry.

ISSUES FOR CHILDREN

Children who have parents or siblings with diabetes should be forewarned in an age-appropriate manner of possible diabetes-related emergencies and how to deal with them.

Children may witness a severe hypoglycemic reaction and may need to provide assistance. It is good to have an emergency plan in place for children for these circumstances. Practice it regularly, just like a fire drill or other emergency plan. Some ways in which children can be prepared for these emergencies are listed in the sidebar below.

Addressing a child's fears about diabetes is important. Many children feel it is inevitable that they will develop diabetes if they see it in their loved ones. It is good to have an open discussion with children and answer their questions about diabetes in simple terms that they can understand. The child's pediatrician or the endocrinologist can also discuss these issues.

CHILDREN'S EMERGENCY READINESS LIST

Here are some ways children can be prepared for an emergency.

▶ Teach them how to call 911

▶ Place a list of emergency phone numbers next to all phones

▶ Identify the locations of items to treat hypoglycemia and which items to use

▶ If the children are old enough, instruct them on where to find and how to use a glucagon kit

---

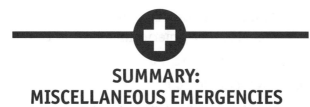

SUMMARY:
MISCELLANEOUS EMERGENCIES

SIGNS OF AN EYE EMERGENCY

▶ Loss of vision

▶ Eye pain

▶ Double or blurred vision

▶ Redness of the eye

▶ Floating or flashing lights

SIGNS OF LOSS OF BLOOD TO THE FEET

▶ Pain

▶ Cool to the touch, lack of warmth

▶ Pale skin, lack of color

▶ No pulse

SIGNS OF A HEART ATTACK

▶ Chest pain

▶ Trouble breathing

▶ Neck, jaw, or arm pain

▶ Back pain

▶ Swelling of the legs

▶ Nausea

SIGNS OF A STROKE

▶ Sudden numbness or weakness in the face, arm, or leg

▶ Confusion

▶ Difficulty speaking or understanding

▶ Trouble seeing

▶ Loss of balance or muscle control

▶ Sudden, severe headache

▶ American Medical ID: www.americanmedical-id.com

▶ Medic Alert: www.medicalert.org

▶ Medic I.D.: www.medic-id.com

▶ Medic ID'S International: www.medicid.com

▶ MedIDs.com: www.medids.com

▶ Vital-ID: www.medicalwristband.com

CHILDREN'S EMERGENCY READINESS LIST

Here are some ways children can be prepared for an emergency.

▶ Teach them how to call 911

▶ Place a list of emergency phone numbers next to all phones

▶ Identify the locations of items to treat hypoglycemia and which items to use

▶ If the children are old enough, instruct them on where to find and how to give a glucagon kit

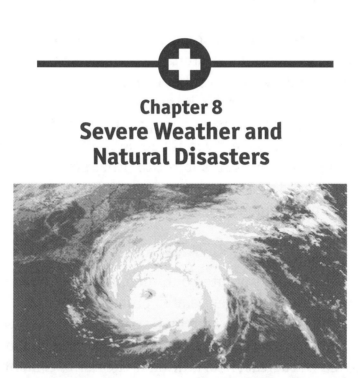

Chapter 8
Severe Weather and
Natural Disasters

An estimated 100,000 people with diabetes were evacuated as a result of Hurricane Katrina in late 2005. Many factors played a role in the aftermath of Hurricane Katrina, directly and indirectly disturbing the diabetes care of those affected by the hurricane. Even for those with the best of circumstances, diabetes management was difficult. Lack of supplies and medicine were obvious problems, but many other unforeseen factors also played a role in disrupting diabetes care—lack of medical records, overcrowding, limited availability of food and water, and lack of medical support (hospitals, clinics, and doctors' offices were closed) all played a role as well. Furthermore, one factor that few foresaw or adequately addressed was depression. The staggering financial losses, loss of personal belongings, and loss of loved ones all contributed to depression, which also makes diabetes control difficult. Although many of the problems with diabetes management could have been prevented, many were unforeseen and difficult to avoid even in the best of circumstances.

Hurricane Katrina and the New Orleans aftermath taught us a great deal about natural disasters and their potential impact on diabetes care. In the very least, they emphasized the importance of planning ahead. It is critical to be prepared for severe weather and natural disasters, so there is no disruption to your diabetes care if something should happen. Even if you do not live in an area that has hurricanes, you are still subject to other potential disasters, such as tornados, floods, blizzards, and earthquakes. You want to be sure that any emergency does not put your health at risk.

PREPARATION

As we have continually pointed out, preparation is the key to preventing a variety of diabetes-related problems under any number of circumstances. As illustrated by Hurricane Katrina, even well-prepared individuals cannot anticipate everything. But, being well prepared will at least help minimize the risk of complications, and being adequately prepared for a natural disaster is certainly no exception. The sidebar on page 104 contains a list of items that should be included in a *disaster preparedness kit*. This kit will contain all of the basic things you may need during a natural disaster (such as a flashlight, batteries, and water), plus diabetes-related items that are in your diabetes supply kit (see page 5).

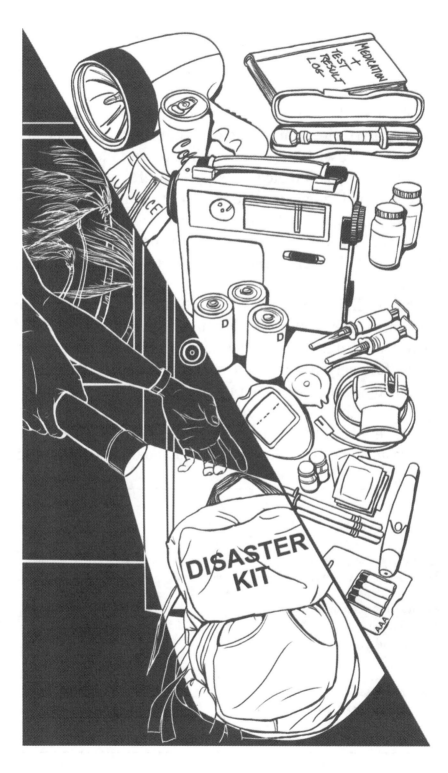

A Few Notes about the Kit

First, this kit is not meant to be assembled and stashed away in your house months in advance. Some of the items can be collected ahead of time (like when hurricane season starts), such as medical history, batteries, water, a sharps container, and some of the diabetes supplies with long or no expiration periods (for example, lancets, test strips, and alcohol wipes). But for many items, it is impractical and inadvisable to do so far in advance. In general, if there is a warning put out to the public of an impending disaster (weather station alerts, radio and television stations, etc.), it is time to collect the remaining items for your disaster preparedness kit.

Second, medicines and certain supplies often cannot be placed in the disaster preparedness kit because of a number of factors (for example, the limited amount allowed by your insurance company). It is therefore very important to make sure your diabetes medicines and supply refills are kept up to date and that the refills are obtained from the pharmacy as often as your insurance company allows. Note also that if you prepare your medical history information in advance, you will also have to update it as information

Basal Rates:
Midnight to 6 AM = 1.1 units/hr
6 AM to 3 PM – 1.0 units/hr
3 PM to 7 PM = 0.9 units/hr
7PM to midnight = 1.1 units/hr
Meal insulin: CHO ratios:
Breakfast 1:8
Lunch and Dinner 1:10
Snacks 1:12
Correction doses:
1 per 25 over 110 (6 AM – 10 PM)
1 per 25 over 130 (10 PM – 6 AM)

changes, such as emergency contact numbers, medical or surgical history, pump settings, and medicine and dose changes.

Third, be sure to periodically check the expiration dates of all supplies and medicines placed in the kit. If the kit is prepared in May or June (the start of hurricane season in some parts of the U.S.) and you ignore it until October, then some of the items may have expired. It is best to check the expiration dates monthly and to establish a system that will remind you to check the supplies. A few common examples include keeping a note taped to the outside of the kit listing the expiration dates, writing a reminder on a wall calendar, or setting up an automated reminder in your computer's calendar.

Last, disaster preparedness kits for people with diabetes are commercially available (search the Internet for "diabetes preparedness kit"). These kits have some of the basic survival items but will not contain any specific medical supplies or medicines that you will need. Even if you choose to purchase a pre-assembled kit, be sure to add medical supplies and medicines that you will need.

MINOR POWER OUTAGES

Minor power outages do not normally last a very long time, so the chances of being evacuated are low. In some cases, however, you may still be forced to leave your home, either because of extreme heat or cold without air conditioning or heat, or for other reasons. If you are able to stay at home during a power outage, there are a few things to keep in mind. This is when having your disaster preparedness kit comes in handy, especially for things like flashlights or lanterns and battery-operated radios.

Drinking plenty of water or other carbohydrate-free drinks is important in preventing dehydration. Keep the house stocked with water ahead of time so you can be sure that plenty of water will be available. Planning ahead can prevent countless problems.

DISASTER PREPAREDNESS KIT

Items with an asterisk (*) can be collected and stored well in advance.

▶ Flashlight and plenty of batteries*

▶ AM/FM radio (with plenty of batteries)*

▶ Bottled water (at least a three-day supply)*

▶ Canned food items

▶ Extra cell phone battery and charger

▶ Small portable cooler with refreezable gel packs
   (do not use dry ice for medicines)*

▶ Diabetes medicines, such as unopened insulin and diabetes pills
   (30-day supply)

▶ Items to treat mild or moderate hypoglycemia

▶ Extra blood glucose meter and batteries (30-day supply)*

▶ Blood glucose test strips (30-day supply)*

▶ Lancets (30-day supply)*

▶ Empty sharps container for used lancets and needles*

▶ Alcohol wipes*

Make sure you have a phone that does not require a separate power supply. Cordless phones need to be plugged into a wall outlet to charge and to dial out, but standard, corded phones do not. Corded phones use the electricity from the telephone wires for power. Keep one of these phones handy in a closet, ready to be used if the power goes out. Cell phones are also great, but their batteries need to be charged, so plan on having an extra charged cell phone battery in your kit. Remember, though, that recharge-able batteries, like those in cell phones, do lose their charge over time, so when you check the expiration dates in your disaster pre-

- Urine ketone strips and blood ketone test strips, if used (30-day supply)*

- Glucagon emergency kits (pack two)

- Insulin syringes and/or pen needles (30-day supply)*

- Insulin pump supplies: plenty of infusion sets, reservoirs, batteries, transparent dressings (if used)

- List of current medicines and their doses*

- List of insulin pump settings (basal rates, meal boluses, and high blood glucose bolus calculations)*

- Pen and paper or logbook to record blood glucose levels*

- Written instructions from your diabetes team for an insulin regimen to use when off an insulin pump (along with the appropriate insulins)*

- List of physicians, their specialties (e.g., cardiologist, kidney doctor, foot doctor, etc.), and their phone numbers*

- List of current and past medical problems, as well as previous surgeries*

- List of medical allergies*

paredness kit, set aside a little time to recharge those cell phone batteries.

If the temperature in the house becomes too hot or too cold and it does not look like power will be restored any time soon, do not hesitate to check into a nearby hotel. This may be a lifesaving decision. Avoiding extreme temperatures is important for good health, especially for the elderly. Plus, insulin may go bad if the house gets too hot.

EVACUATIONS

Being away from home for an extended period can be stressful. No one likes to be in unfamiliar surroundings, particularly if you have been forced out of your home because of severe weather or a natural disaster. This is especially true if you are forced to stay at a shelter. Here are a few important points if you have to stay in a shelter or are otherwise away from home.

Be sure someone else knows that you have diabetes. Those in charge of the shelter should know in case a diabetes emergency develops. Also, make sure you wear your medical alert ID. If you don't have one, it is important to get one (see page 95).

Be sure to check your blood glucose levels frequently. The stress of the situation may cause your blood glucose levels to rise. However, if you are eating less food than usual, your blood glucose levels may be lower. If you find that your blood glucose levels are consistently high or low, insulin adjustments may be needed. Contact your diabetes team for guidance.

Remember that opened vials of insulin and insulin pens in use can be safely stored at room temperature. There is no need to keep them in a cooler, although unopened vials or pens/cartridges are better kept in a refrigerator or cooler. Furthermore, insulin should not be exposed to excessive heat or cold temperatures. Keeping your insulin at a regulated temperature will prevent it from going bad. Also, be sure to look at your insulins before using them. Regular insulin, rapid-acting insulins (insulin lispro [Humalog], insulin aspart [NovoLog], and insulin glulisine [Apidra]), and long-acting insulins (insulin glargine [Lantus] and insulin detemir [Levemir]) should be crystal clear. If these insulins are cloudy, thick, or contain particles, throw them away. Premixed and NPH insulins, although used less frequently than the ones previously mentioned, are supposed to be cloudy but should not have any particles visible in the insulin solution. Last, although it is best to avoid reusing insulin syringes or pen needles, it may become necessary to do this in an emergency situation.

Drink plenty of water. Preventing dehydration is very important. Note that if your blood glucose levels are high, you are at greater risk of dehydration and problems related to dehydration, such as DKA.

Preventing hypoglycemia is very important, especially if you take insulin or use some types of diabetes pills. This is why your disaster preparedness kit should be stocked with carbohydrate-containing foods to treat hypoglycemia. In some situations, the best way to prevent hypoglycemia is to aim for slightly higher sugar levels than usual.

CONCLUSION

No matter where you live, there is the chance that you will have to deal with extreme and severe weather or other natural disasters. Experience has taught us that preparing for these uncommon—but *real*—emergencies is the single most important way to reduce the chances that your health will be put in danger. We can take one positive note from Hurricane Katrina: it raised awareness about the many potential problems that people with diabetes (or any other chronic health condition) and their family members face when there is severe weather or a natural disaster.

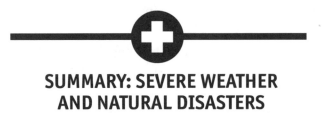

SUMMARY: SEVERE WEATHER AND NATURAL DISASTERS

DISASTER PREPAREDNESS KIT

Items with an asterisk (*) can be collected and stored well in advance.

- Flashlight and plenty of batteries*
- AM/FM radio (with plenty of batteries)*
- Bottled water (at least a three-day supply)*
- Canned food items
- Extra cell phone battery and charger
- Small portable cooler with refreezable gel packs (do not use dry ice for medicines)*
- Diabetes medicines, such as unopened insulin and diabetes pills (30-day supply)
- Items to treat mild or moderate hypoglycemia
- Extra blood glucose meter and batteries (30-day supply)*
- Blood glucose test strips (30-day supply)*
- Lancets (30-day supply)*

- Empty sharps container for used lancets and needles*
- Alcohol wipes*
- Urine ketone strips and blood ketone test strips, if used (30-day supply)*
- Glucagon emergency kits (pack two)
- Insulin syringes and/or pen needles (30-day supply)*
- Insulin pump supplies: plenty of infusion sets, reservoirs, batteries, transparent dressings (if used)
- List of current medicines and their doses*
- List of insulin pump settings (basal rates, meal boluses, and high blood glucose bolus calculations)*
- Pen and paper or logbook to record blood glucose levels*
- Written instructions from your diabetes team for an insulin regimen to use when off an insulin pump (along with the appropriate insulins)*
- List of physicians, their specialties (e.g., cardiologist, kidney doctor, foot doctor, etc.), and their phone numbers*
- List of current and past medical problems, as well as previous surgeries*
- List of medical allergies*

TIPS FOR EVACUATIONS

- Be sure someone else knows you have diabetes.
- Wear your medical ID.
- Check your blood glucose levels frequently.
- Opened vials of insulin and insulin pens in use can be safely stored at room temperature for up to one month after the vial is opened; save the space in your cooler for other items.
- Insulin should not be exposed to extreme temperatures.
- Look at the insulins before each use. Regular, rapid-acting, and long-acting insulins should be crystal clear.

▶ Although it is best to avoid reusing insulin syringes or pen needles, it may become necessary to do this.

▶ Try to drink plenty of water. Preventing dehydration is important.

▶ Have juice or other sources of carbohydrate available to treat hypoglycemia.

▶ Your blood glucose target may have to be adjusted, aiming for slightly higher levels than normal in order to prevent hypoglycemia.

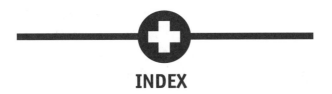

INDEX

cornea, 88–89. *See also* eyes
cranial nerve palsies, 90

D

daycare, 6
dehydration, 9, 103, 107, 109. *See also* diabetic ketoacidosis (DKA)
dentists. *See* medical team
depression, 59, 61–68, 100
diabetes
    supply kit, 3–10, 17, 47, 55–56, 71, 100–102. *See also* insulin pump therapy; supplies; travel
    type 1, 1, 39, 45, 63
    type 2, 1, 38–39, 45, 63
diabetic ketoacidosis (DKA), 38–39, 42–44, 46. *See also* ketones
diabetic neuropathy. *See* neuropathy
diabetic retinopathy. *See* retinopathy
diarrhea, 33, 42, 44. *See also* illness; sick day supplies
dining out, 78, 84
disaster preparedness kit, 99–109
disc, 88
doctors. *See* medical team
drug abuse, 64

E

electrolytes, 33–34, 43
emergency

eyes, 87–90, 97
feet, 91–92, 97
miscellaneous, 87
room, 42, 44
types of, 1–2
emotions, 59, 65
evacuations, 106–107, 109–110
exercise, 13, 15, 19–22, 28, 64
expiration dates, 6, 17, 103
eye doctor. *See* medical team
eyes, 87–90, 97

F

feet, 91–92, 97
fever, 33. *See also* illness; sick day supplies
flu, 42, 44. *See also* illness; sick day supplies
fluids, 33–35, 41–43, 78, 81, 103–104, 107. *See also* dehydration
food, 13, 23–25, 64, 75, 78
fovea, 88
frustration, 59

G

gastroparesis, 36
glaucoma, 87, 90
glimepiride, 14
glipizide, 14
glucagon, 6, 17–18, 28, 71, 78, 96
glucose, 6, 33–34. *See also* blood glucose levels; carbohydrates
glyburide, 13

H

heart attack, 92–93, 97
heart problems, 63, 92–93. *See also*
    heart attack
high blood pressure, 63
hormones, 14, 17, 31, 39
hospital, 42, 44
Hurricane Katrina, 99–100
hyperglycemia, 42
hypertension. *See* high blood
    pressure
hypoglycemia
    airport security, 75–76, 83–84
    and alcohol, 14, 22–24
    causes of, 13–14, 27
    children's emergency readiness
        list, 96, 98
    continuous glucose monitors, 26
    and depression, 64
    diabetes supply kit, 5–6, 9
    disaster preparedness kit, 104,
        108
    evacuations, 107
    and exercise, 15, 19–22, 27–28
    food related, 23–25
    nighttime, 19, 54
    overtreatment, 15–16
    prevention, 11–12, 19, 24
    risk, 8, 10
    Rule of 15, 17, 27–28
    severe, 16–17
    support team, 11
    symptoms, 12, 15, 27
    and travel, 78, 84
    treatment, 13–18
    warning signs, 8, 10, 12

I

identification, medical alert,
    94–96, 98, 106
illness, 8–10, 23–24, 31–44.
    See also alcohol; sick day
    supplies
infants, 13, 17–18, 34
injections, 7–8, 24–25, 29, 40–41,
    46, 52–57, 73, 81, 86
insulin
    aspart, 26, 41, 48
    delivery, interrupted, 56
    detemir, 26, 40, 53–55, 57, 73
    and diabetic ketoacidosis
        (DKA), 38–39
    dosages, 7–8, 24–26, 31–32,
        36–37, 40–41, 47, 49, 51–57,
        80–81, 86
    errors, 25–26
    and exercise, 19–22, 28
    function of, 38–40
    glargine, 26, 40, 53–54, 57, 73
    glulisine, 26, 41, 48
    and hypoglycemia, 10, 19
    injections, 7–8, 40–41
    lispro, 26, 41, 48
    long-acting, 26, 40–41, 47,
        53–54, 57, 73
    NPH, 25, 41
    production, 36–37
    rapid-acting, 26, 41, 48, 52–53,
        55, 57
    resistance, 31–33, 38
    short-acting, 73
    storage, 6, 106–107
    supply, 7–8, 10

OTHER TITLES FROM THE
AMERICAN DIABETES ASSOCIATION

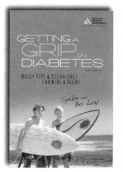

Getting a Grip on Diabetes, 2nd Edition
by Spike Nasmyth Loy and Bo Nasmyth Loy
For children learning to navigate the world of type 1 diabetes comes this revised guide from the people who have firsthand experience. Spike and Bo, who both have had type 1 diabetes since they were children, teach kids of all ages everything they need to know about managing diabetes, including recognizing hypoglycemia, going to college, and traveling safely.
Order no. 4909-02; Price $14.95

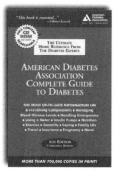

American Diabetes Association
Complete Guide to Diabetes, 4th Edition
by American Diabetes Association
Have all the tips and information on diabetes that you need close at hand. The world's largest collection of diabetes self-care tips, techniques, and tricks for solving diabetes-related problems is back in its fourth edition, and it's bigger and better than ever before.
Order no. 4809-04; New low price $19.95

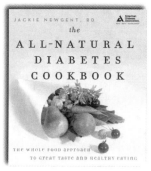

The All-Natural Diabetes Cookbook:
The Whole Food Approach to
Great Taste and Healthy Eating
by Jackie Newgent, RD
Instead of relying on artificial sweeteners or not-so-real substitutions to reduce calories, sugar, and fat, *The All-Natural Diabetes Cookbook* takes a different approach, focusing on naturally delicious fresh foods and whole-food ingredients to create fantastic meals that deliver amazing taste and well-rounded nutrition. And absolutely nothing is artificial.
Order no. 4663-01; Price $18.95

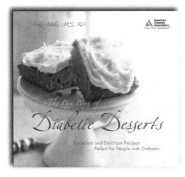

The Big Book of Diabetic Desserts
by Jackie Mills, MS, RD
This first-ever collection of guilty pleasures proves that people with diabetes never have to say no to dessert again. Packed with familiar favorites and some delicious new surprises, *The Big Book of Diabetic Desserts* has more than 150 tantalizing treats that will satisfy any sweet tooth.

Order no. 4664-01; Price $18.95

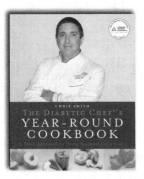

The Diabetic Chef's Year-Round Cookbook
by Chris Smith, The Diabetic Chef
Are you tired of uninspired, bland meals? Then you're ready for the creative dishes from The Diabetic Chef. Take advantage of seasonal foods available from month to month and enjoy a year of amazing, market-fresh meals. With *The Diabetic Chef's Year-Round Cookbook*, you'll enjoy perfect hors d'oeuvres to start off a dinner party and find the best entrees to delight your family on a weeknight.

Order no. 4667-01; Price 19.95

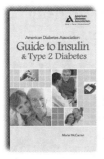

American Diabetes Association Guide to Insulin & Type 2 Diabetes
by Marie McCarren
Insulin is the most powerful tool available for managing diabetes when pills, exercise, and a careful diet are no longer enough. *The American Diabetes Association Guide to Insulin & Type 2 Diabetes* gives you the complete information on insulin plans you need and gives you advice from the experts: people with diabetes who use insulin.

Order no. 5022-01; Price $12.95

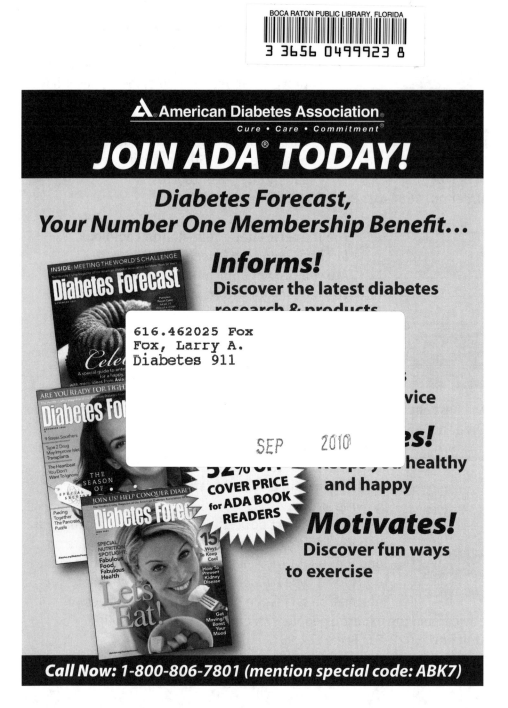